A BOLD PERSPECTIVE

Tina Marie Fuller and Rashon Fuller

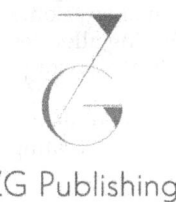

ZG Publishing

A Bold Perspective
Copyright © 2015
by Tina Marie Fuller and Rashon Fuller

All rights reserved. No part of this book may be used, reproduced, scanned or distributed in print, electronic form or in any manner whatsoever without the written permission of the Publisher is illegal and punishable by law.
Please purchase only authorized print and electronic editions. Please do not participate in or encourage piracy of copyrighted material. Your support of the author's rights is appreciated.

For information visit:
www.Soliberating.com

Tina Marie Fuller and Rashon Fuller
A Bold Perspective

Printed in the United States of America

ISBN: 978-0-9963425-0-6 (Paperback)
978-0-9963425-1-3 (eBook)

Publisher – ZG Publishing

Cover Design – Madison McClintock
www.madisonjmcclintock.com

Ish Holmes
www.ishholmes.com

Natasha
C8M Creative Team

Disclaimer: The author and the publisher of this book does not dispense medical advice or dictate the use of any technique as a form of treatment for physical, emotional, mental or medical issues without the advice of a physician, either directly or indirectly. A Bold Perspective is only offering information to assist in your journey for mental, spiritual, emotional, and physical wellness.
We do not warrant that the use of recipes in this book will necessarily aid in the prevention or treatment of any disease. We disclaim any liability, loss, or risk, personal or otherwise incurred as a consequence, directly or indirectly of the use and application of any content in this book.
For those with special needs including allergies or health problems please contact your medical advisor prior to use.

ZG Publishing
www.Soliberating.com
Copyright © 2015

All rights reserved.

A BOLD PERSPECTIVE

BOLD

- adjective

1. not hesitating or fearful in the face of actual or possible danger or rebuff.
2. necessitating courage and daring.
3. beyond the usual limits of conventional thought or action.

PERSPECTIVE

- noun

1. mental view or prospect.

A BOLD PERSPECTIVE

A FULLER Contribution to Life and Love.

May you discover Personal Liberation in your Mind, Body, and Spirit.

CONTENTS

DEDICATIONS ix
INTRODUCTION 1
SECTION 1: GLORY AND BLUES ....
INCEPTION 7
THE WEEKEND 21
CAST DOWN 25
LIVE ON 35
EXERTION 45
ALTERATION 51
LIFE AS IT WAS 63
NOTEBOOK 77
SECOND CHANCE 79
UNTITLED 87
BREAKING OF DAY 93
PROGRESSION 95
RE-WRITING THE PAST 101
PERSONAL LIBERATION 105
THE RIGHT FUTURE 117
TEAM FULLER 121
LOVE LETTERS 129

SECTION 2: LIFE IN ABUNDANCE 137

INTRODUCTION 139

POWER OF LOVE 143

GENESIS 149

CREATE YOUR PAUSE 153

INSTAGRAM vs. REALITY 155

THE SELFIE 157

THE BEAUTIFUL STRUGGLE 159

FITNESS 165

SECTION 3: GOC 171

GENESIS OF CHANGE aka GOC 173

BACK TO THE BASICS 177

THE JOURNEY 187

WELCOME TO GENESIS OF CHANGE! 203

MISSION COMPLETE 243

ACKNOWLEDGEMENTS 249

REFERENCES 251

DEDICATION

To a perfect God, who never wastes an EXPERIENCE.

To the essence of this LITTLE BOY... *my son Kevin.*

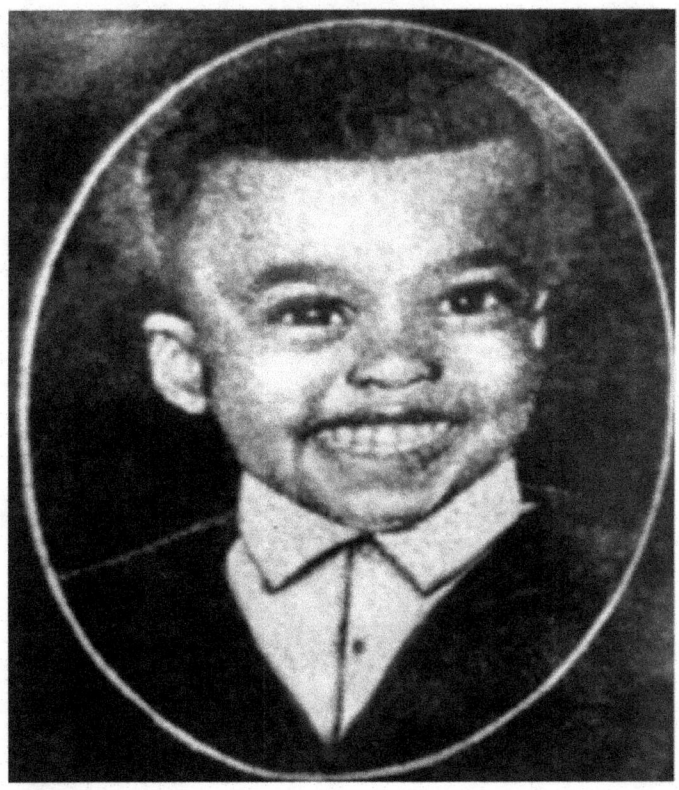

And to the memory of my Uncle Tyrone Dale, a kind soul, who loved to read.

INTRODUCTION

At the onset of tragedy, I made myself a promise. If God allowed me my footing and gave me the strength to walk on, then I would. Every morning I had breath and mobility, so I got up… and I journeyed on. However, after 16 years of motion and anguish, I realized that I had reached my breaking point. If I woke on tomorrow and if my current situation was still the same, that day would be day one of a grave depression.

Moments later a phone call altered my course. A woman whom I did not know, ignited a spark as she spoke words of assurance into my life. "God said that he has not forgotten about you. He is going to restore you, *-BUT first you must share your story."* I wish that I could say with excitement and joy I got straight to writing my story, but no! I had no interest in exposing my hurts, my disappointments, and my brokenness on a public platform; however I chose to trust the process.

Nevertheless, NOT MY WILL, BUT THINE, BE DONE. -Luke 22:42

I'm sure that we have all heard the phrase "life is what you make it." But, that philosophy is not always true. At times with no warning calamity will come along and take all the sunshine away in 0.1 seconds flat. Picture the perfect day…the sun is blazing, and the sky is so very blue, not one cloud in sight then out of nowhere…BOOM… the storms of life have rushed in like a flood, destroying everything in its path. Now we find ourselves devastated, desolated, and totally depleted.

Life as we once knew it no longer exists. We are left with the doom and gloom of massive clouds filled with hurt and responsibilities: working, paying bills, taking care of our families, tormenting memories of what happened and how life used to be before "IT" happened. We are left toting mental, emotional, spiritual and physical woes, all while pondering over and over again what we could have been done differently or we disassociate ourselves; altogether avoiding the agony. In this state of being we aren't living, we're just existing, mission survival mode.

But there is hope and the answer lies within us! Collectively and individually despite the opposition we must fight *Pro-Life*. We weren't designed to succumb to our problems. We were designed to conquer! Come travel along and together let's explore the Why (our calling) and Reason (our purpose) for this thing called life!

I don't know about you but life has taught me a lesson or two. I don't tread the land empty handed. I carry my two edged sword and my boom box. One end of my sword has the word of God. The other end is like that old school pen. You know the one with the four different color tips—blue, black, red and green. Instead of ink my sword has courage which allows me to face my fears; determination that won't allow me to quit on myself; a light so in my midnight hour I can see my way. And my e`pee, aka (also known) as my blade, which cuts the throat of the adversary.

I hope that YOU will grab your sword too. You'll need it; but don't sweat it. We got your back! Me and my Ace (husband Rashon) we got you!

The journey won't be easy. From this view the road may look straight, but ahead there are winding roads ahead where our deepest fears and secrets are exposed. At times we will reach our breaking point, but don't worry. Even then, we will persevere, if we faint not. At that point, God will meet us there like he always does and he will give us strength to complete the journey. Oh yeah, about my boom box…it's an internal box that's based in the center of my heart. I've been on this road for quite a while and what I have learned is you've got to find your song. I have several! At times life leaves me at a total loss for words and in those moments, my soul sings and I am encouraged to carry on.

WAIT!

Grab your backpack. You've got to have a *journal*, a *pen* and a *mirror*.

Previously, I mentioned that life is not always what you make it. HOWEVER, we do possess the power to change and mold our outcome.

Okay, God Here I go.

I hear and I obey.

~Tina Marie aka TM

A BOLD PERSPECTIVE

ROLL CALL

I am Here!
The Real ME; the one God created me to be.
I have FINALLY rose!

And I Am Here!

Cypher to my Secrets.
Shalom to my Fears.
There's a Story to be told,
And I **AM HERE**!!!
ROLL CALL…
I AM HERE!

TM.

Now, I need to preface this…I'm about to pull back the layers and go below the surface while sharing MY STORY.

If you did NOT read the introduction GO BACK<<<

SECTION 1
GLORY AND BLUES

CHAPTER 1

INCEPTION

I walked into the clinic and went to the receptionist desk.

"Hi. I am here to take the test." I said.

"Sure." The receptionist replied. "Sign in, fill out this form, then have a seat in the waiting area. Your name will be called soon. After three o'clock, you can call in for your test results."

After taking the test, time did what it never does: it stood still. Every second felt like minutes. Every minute felt like an hour. When the clock finally struck 3 o'clock, I grabbed the phone and swiftly dialed the number. Now, by this point I had all seven digits memorized.

As the phone rang my stomach quivered with nervousness. Then suddenly, they answered, "Hello, thank you for calling Kaiser how may I help you?"

"Hi. My name is Tina Lindsey. I came in today for a test and I'm calling for the results."

"Please hold." The receptionist replied.

The silence was nerve-wrecking. My breathing became scattered, and I felt like I was going to have an asthma attack. Each millisecond of silence was like a pounding drum because my heart felt like it was going to jump out of my chest.

Then finally, she returned. "Tina?"

"Yes!" I answered.

"Your results came back positive."

"POSITIVE? Are you sure?" I asked.

"Yes. Positive." She repeated.

I dropped the receiver and just stood there in shock.

"OH MY GOD! This cannot be... not to me!"

But deep down inside, I knew it. I had never been more than 2 days late and at this point I was over 2 weeks late. I was immediately afraid. There was no way I could tell my parents I was pregnant. They would kill me. On second thought... no way is Mylon going to believe I'm pregnant with his child.

Let's go back so I can explain...

At school rumors began to surface that Mylon and Kacie were talking. You know, like they were about to become an item. *That kind of talking...* I asked Mylon were the rumors true. He gave a whole song and dance about how that was a lie. I wanted to believe him, but I decided to keep my eyes and my ears open.

Wait! *Let's go back even further; this story needs a few more details.*

It seemed like it all started the first day of middle school. I was already nervous about being at a big new school with hundreds of students. My school day went from having two teachers to six teachers and the responsibility of managing a locker, a ton of books and peer pressure, was pretty overwhelming. As if that wasn't enough, one day while standing at my locker a girl began to talk slick to me. I was totally intimidated. Until that moment I had never seen her before, but quickly I learned that her name was Kacie and she was a 7th grader. Kacie was twice my size, well not in height but certainly in width. She was always with a clique of friends (no less than three to five at any given time). From our first encounter, whenever she saw me she was sure to make some sly remark.

This foolishness went on for months until one day our paths crossed on the way to class. I was going up the steps as she was coming down. It was just the two of us, and she didn't say one word. She only rolled her eyes initially. However, once she got to the bottom of the steps she made her usual sly remark. After that, it was on! It was evident that her shenanigans were for the attention she would get from an audience. I made a choice to no longer be a victim to her bullying. Starting that day, every dialogue with her was a heated exchange. To my surprise, her friends never got involved either. They stood on the sidelines during our verbal spars.

The exchanges continued throughout all of sixth grade. Kacie was the bully type, but I learned firsthand that bullies thrive on fear, and I was no longer afraid. By the time seventh grade rolled around we didn't say much to each other. As the seventh grade school year came to an end I was super excited for two reasons, next year I would be an eighth grader and no more Kacie for an entire year! Within a day or so, my joy shifted as word quickly spread that she had failed 8th grade and would be repeating it. All summer long I hoped that it was just a rumor, but as 8th grade rolled around, the rumors proved to be true. Like 7th grade, we didn't say much to one another, but our hatred for each other spoke volumes.

By the time we entered high school, I rarely saw her. She was out of sight and completely out of my mind! But when our paths did cross, the flaring of my nostrils was a clear indicator that I still hated her.

One day while running super late to first period, I was praying that my teacher would let me in class and not send me to detention. As I turned the final corner, I saw them with my own two eyes. Mylon wasn't just standing at Kacie's locker. He was leaning in on her locker with his left leg over his right. His body's disposition suggested he was spitting some cold game. The look in his face when he saw me was as if he had seen a ghost. I didn't say one word. He didn't deserve to hear my voice. In that moment, we had a speechless breakup. There was nothing to be said. He couldn't lie his way out of this one. He knew how I felt about her. He didn't just play me. What he did was unforgivable and I was done.

The school year ended as the summer of 1994 began, but all I could think about was the summer of 1993. I had the time of my life. I thought about all the times Chiron, Rudah and I hung out with Mylon, Evan, and Mason. Gordon Park was our spot. A year later Chiron and Evan were still together, and so were Rudah and Mason. I was left feeling like the odd ball. Our breakup was still fresh. Every song on the radio reminded me of when we were together. As hard as it was, I stayed strong. I refused to call him and eventually after receiving my cold shoulder he stopped calling me.

After a few months of no communication, I got a phone call one day. Honestly, the moment I heard his voice on the other end my summer felt complete, I totally melted. He apologized and told me how he messed up. He professed his love for me amongst a host of other sweet nothings. I had managed to reject all his advances until he told me that Chiron and Evan were hanging out that night. He asked if I wanted to hang out too… "Ya know, like old times?" I couldn't resist. How could I? Chiron was my absolute favorite cousin and I was missing Mylon like crazy!

We hung out at the park. We laughed, joked, and listened to music from Evan's car stereo. Later that evening, I ended up at Mylon's house and we chilled on his front porch. Eventually he invited me in the house to watch TV, and before I knew it one thing lead to another. At the start of penetration I asked him to stop and he did. Mylon was my first *real* boyfriend. Prior to our breakup, we were together for a year and truthfully I was still in love with him, but his actions were foul. I felt that getting back together with him was *devaluing* myself, even if he was sincerely sorrowful. I explained my position and he acknowledged it while offering up another apology for his prior actions. He expressed how he wished that he could take back what he had done, but reality doesn't work that way and we both knew that. As we walked out of his front door, I knew that I would never cross that threshold again. Mylon escorted me back home and that was the last of us.

Surrounding these circumstances, how could I call him now and tell him and expect for him to believe it! Heck, I couldn't believe it myself and I had a doctor's test to confirm it. But, I had to call him, so I did.

Even though, I knew it was him that answered the phone. I still started with Hello, may I speak to Mylon. I just needed a few extra seconds to gather myself.

He was cool as a cucumber. "Hey! Whuz up Tina! You know this me."

My voice was trembling. I could barely speak. After a moment of hesitation, I spewed it out.

"I am pregnant."

"Pregnant? Yeah right!" was his first response.

But I guess that he could tell by the tone of my voice that I was serious. He followed with, "How do you know?"

"I went to Kaiser today." I replied.

There was total silence on both ends of the phone. Finally, after a few minutes....

He asked "What do you want to do?"

"Well right now I'm over my Aunt Jewel's house and I'm going to see if she can take me to get an abortion. We can just use Chiron's birth certificate." I had a plan, and keeping this baby was not a part of it.

"Is that what you want to do? Get an abortion?" He asked compassionately.

I quickly responded, "Yes! I'm not ready for a baby."

Then he said, "Okay. After you talk to Mrs. J, call me back and let me know what I need to do."

"Okay I'll call you right back!"

I hung up the phone and went downstairs to talk to Auntie Jewel and Chiron. A few minutes later I call him back.

"Hello?"

"Yeah, it's me," I replied.

She said no.

I tried to explain my situation and my plan to Auntie Jewel and Chiron. Before I could finish, Chiron blared out "This isn't a good idea! Your parents need to know what's going on in case something goes wrong."

"I can't believe I'm pregnant and I can't believe they told me no to an abortion. My parents are going to kill me!"

I continued on as Mylon tried to calm me down but nothing worked. I was a nervous wreck. That evening Auntie Jewel, Chiron and I had a discussion at the kitchen table on how to tell my parents. The next evening Auntie Jewel dropped me off at home, which was a little less than a three mile drive. We both lived in Cleveland Heights, but on opposite ends of the suburb. During the entire ride, my Aunt who is my mom's sister kept saying, "Tina your mom is not going to kill you. You will be okay. If you need me or your Uncle Phil to come back and get you, just call me."

Back in my bedroom, I paced the floor. My thoughts were racing, and I decided I needed an ally.

"Kisha, come here," I whispered to my sister, who was two years my senior.

"W H A T? And, why are you whispering?" she asked as she entered my room.

"Shhhhh... DANG! I'm trying to tell you something. I just found out that

I'm pregnant, and I'm about to tell mommy and daddy."

"Really?

You are pregnant? You're about to tell them now?" she asked.

"Yes," I replied.

"Then I'm about to go to over my friend Leah's house because I don't want any parts of this.

Good Luck!" Kisha said.

As soon as she shut the back door the telephone rang. I knew it was time to execute the plan.

A few minutes later I heard my father say, "I'll be back in a little bit. I'm about to take a ride." Then the back door shut for a second time.

I paced and I paced. Then I paced a little while longer until I finally forced myself outside my bedroom's threshold. At first, I was frozen in the hallway. After a few minutes, I reluctantly stepped into my parents' room.

"Hey. What's up Tina?" My mother asked.

With each second of hesitation, my mother looked immensely concerned. It was as if she knew what I was about to say, but at the same time she hoped I didn't say it...

"I have something to tell you. Uncle Phil just picked dad up so I could tell you by myself, and he is going to tell him what I am about to share."

"I am… pregnant."

All at once her facial expression showed disappointment, rage, and shock. I could see that she was angry.

"I'm sorry. I didn't mean to get pregnant." I tried to explain. As soon as those words parted my lips, the back door slammed.

I was scared to death…

Each footstep sounded as if Goliath had entered our house. I couldn't hold my head up anymore and I began to tremble. In total despair I kept my head down as I cried.

"T I N A! Come Here!"

I looked up to find him standing in the doorway with his arms stretched wide. In my father's arms, I wept.

About five minutes later, he let me go. We both wiped our tears, as I began to plead. "I don't want to keep this baby. Please let me get an abortion."

"Well, Tina if you didn't want a baby you shouldn't have gotten yourself pregnant. You won't be getting an abortion" my father said.

"Can I give the baby up for adoption?" I asked.

"Adoption? No. Nobody gave you up for adoption." He replied.

"There will be NO abortion. NO adoption. " My father said.

"But what about school?" I asked as I tried to sway his decision.

"You'll finish school. You just made life tough on yourself, but as a family we will get through this together."

"Let me guess. Mylon?" My mother asked.

Yes. I answered.

The next day arrangements were made for all of us to have a sit down, including Mylon and his mother. We'd both met each other's parents before. But, our parents had never formally met. Our mothers had one awkward exchange that involved the new technological advancement of Caller ID. Mylon tried to tell me about it, but I didn't believe him. At the time, it was like some space age idea I'd seen on TV. Mylon's mother worked second shift. One day, I had called and she told me Mylon was on punishment and couldn't accept phone calls for a week. However, with her work schedule we would always talk. This one particular evening it was almost 10pm, and he hadn't called since that morning. This should've been a sign but it didn't register. So, I called him. The phone rang twice then she answered.

"Hello?"

Out of panic, I hung up. Immediately our house phone rang. I snatched it up on the first ring before my parents could answer. They were in the next room and the cordless phone was on the bookshelf next to my mom.

"Hello? Did you just call here and hang up on me?" she asked.

I tried to whisper my lie. "NO Ma'am."

Then she said, "You know what, let me speak with your mother."

From the kitchen with shame and guilt in my voice, I said, "Mom, telephone..."

Five minutes later I heard the receiver hit the base followed by my mom laughing.

She teased, "I bet you won't hang up on her no more! We will be getting a Caller ID too. I'm so sick of y'all's friends doing the same thing to me."

Up until now, that was the first and last time our parents had communicated.

The next morning as I was in my bedroom, I heard the doorbell ring and a few moments later my mom called my name. As I came to the living room, Ms. Lacy was alone.

My mom asked the first question. "So, where is Mylon?"

"I'm sorry Val. He didn't want to come" Ms. Lacy replied.

"Well, my daughter is pregnant. What is he saying about all of this?" my mom asked.

"We talked for quite a while and he said if Tina says this is his child, then it is. So, we are on board." Ms. Lacy Replied.

For me that was a great relief. I was very proud of Mylon's response and I couldn't blame him for not coming to this meeting. I didn't want to be at the meeting either, but I had NO choice.

After Ms. Lacy left I realized that I made it through my two biggest fears: I was still alive and Mylon didn't deny this baby. Yet, here I was 16-years-old and stuck in a pregnant woman's body and respectfully with no choice. I didn't set out to become a teenage mom. Who would? AND Why? But on the same token… I didn't practice safe sex either. Prior to that moment, I had never thought much about pregnancy. I guess I thought I was too young or altogether invincible, but on second thought who could get pregnant from 5 seconds of partial penetration?"

I was pregnant, miserable and embarrassed. I would cringe when people would attempt to touch my stomach. Daily I tried to wish all of this away, but daily it remained. Truth is, I could have gone and had an abortion anyways. I had older friends who would have allowed me to use their IDs but I could still hear Chiron saying "what if something goes wrong," and after my parents decision, I dared not to disobey.

Straight away, I got a job at the Old Country Buffet. I worked Monday – Friday, normally from 11 to close, which meant about 10 p.m. Some nights we didn't finish cleaning until almost midnight. Between the pregnancy and the job, I was so tired. One late night after my shift, as I plopped myself down inside the car with my dad, he said, "you really don't have to work this job. Besides school is around the corner and I would prefer for you to focus on that." About a week later, which was one week before school started, I resigned.

After finding out that I was pregnant, I enrolled into the vocational cosmetology program that my school offered. It seemed ideal for me. I would graduate high school with my diploma and 1500 cosmetology hours. I would only have to pass the state board exam and I would be a licensed stylist.

The summer had ended and school was back in. Everything was different. Before pregnancy, I was a C student at best. My favorite part of school was all things social… friends, cheerleading, and the games. But this school year, I was focused. I was now an A, B student who actually studied and did her homework.

None of the conversations made it my way, but I am sure that our situation was the forefront of massive gossip and rightfully so. Kacie and myself returned back to school both pregnant by Mylon. To add spice to the gossip, he had a new girlfriend her name was Alicia and we all went to the same school, Cleveland Heights High. This was so not atypical for our uppity suburban school.

Kacie and I still didn't see each other much. I had cosmetology for most of the day and it was in another building. For that matter, I didn't see Mylon much either. But it was still quite awkward. Within a few months, Kacie and Mylon both dropped out of school. After that my school days became very peaceful.

One day while in cosmetology class, there was a knock on the door. My teacher stepped out into the hall to meet with the woman at the door. Seconds later, she stuck her head back in the classroom. "Tina may I see you?"

"Me?" I asked.

She nodded "Yes."

Once I got into the hall, she introduced me to the lady. "Tina, this is Mrs. Warren. She teaches a parenting class over at the high school, and I have signed you up for her class."

A BOLD PERSPECTIVE

"What? I don't have time in my schedule to take her class. Cosmetology only allows an additional three courses, and I'm already taking algebra, English, and history." I said.

Mrs. Warren replied, "I have already had the principle drop your history class. You didn't need another history credit. So, your sixth period class is now with me."

I was fuming. My cosmetology teacher had overstepped her boundaries and was violating my rights. My life seemed to be dictated by everyone else's decisions. I was pregnant and didn't want to be. Now I was being forced to take a parenting class. At the end of class, I gave my teacher a piece of my mind and she gave me a piece of hers, too. I spent the next two days in detention, and needless to say my parents had to have a conference with the administrators at the school before I could return to my cosmetology class.

On the third day, I was allowed back into class. But first, I had to have a meeting with the junior and senior cosmetology teachers, Mrs Kirkland and Mrs. Pollard. I was so upset. In the meeting I was full of attitude and rage as I still spoke my mind about my rights being violated.

The first day of the parenting class wasn't so bad. It was composed of a caring teacher and one dozen moms and expecting moms. After a few weeks, I grew to really enjoy the class. We had weekly guests who taught us about credit, balancing finances, how to make quick and easy meals, etc. One of the perks of the class was ten free bus passes per week. My mom took me to school every day. Going home, I would either have my mom pick me up from school or I would walk home with Chiron and my mom would picked me from there later that evening. So, I sold my passes. Another perk of the class was financial assistance with daycare fees. Within a month I truly appreciated Mrs. Kirkland's wisdom...

One day after a long and exhausting day at school, I climbed into my parents' bed. I was suddenly awakened by severe pains. I made my way downstairs and told my mom what I was experiencing. She said, "Grab your bag. You're in labor!"

Off to the hospital we went. As she drove, I removed my seat belt in hopes to find comfort. It didn't work. Before I knew it, I was on my knees on the car floor. I could hear mom saying, "Tina you have to get up, and how did you get down there?" But I couldn't get up. I was in so much pain. I have zero tolerance for pain, so I was suffering.

When we arrived at the hospital, I was placed in a wheel chair and rolled into the labor and delivery room. I immediately asked for an epidural. After the doctor checked me, she declined the epidural. I wasn't dilated enough. After about an hour, I asked again and was denied for a second time. I told the doctor "I couldn't take the pain anymore, and I needed to go home." The painful contractions, beeping machines, poking and prodding, and cords attached to my body was way too much. I was done!

My mom laughed. "Tina! You can't go anywhere until you have this baby."

"Can I go for a walk? I can't just lay in pain like this."

"Sure," the doctor replied. "That will help the baby to come down."

As I slumbered down the halls, my cousin Jae who was also good friends with Mylon had arrived. He was excited that a new baby boy was being born into our family of chiefly girls. Hours later, I received an epidural and it was time to push.

After two hours of pushing, BABY KEVIN ARRIVED!

It was love at first sight! He was my son and I was his mother. I held him in my arms and stared into his face for hours. He had my eyes, my nose, my bottom lip (full) and his father's top lip (thin) and his eyebrows.

This baby gave me a sense of purpose. One I hadn't had until that moment. I was determined to not just get by in life, but to excel. Even though I was only 17 and in the eleventh grade myself, I needed to show this kid that no matter what obstacles life presented…with focus, effort and God, he could excel. Prior to that moment, I had not thought much about college. But now, we were going. I was going after high school and so was he. I realized *leading by example* was *far more powerful* than directing through advice.

For the three-day stay, we had nonstop guests: family, friends, nurses and other new moms. On the last day of our hospital stay, a woman walked into the room.

"May I see your baby because he seems to be the talk of the hospital?" As she looked at him, while my mom held him in her arms, she said, "Well, he is beautiful!" Then she asked me, "Did it hurt?"

"Uummm, seriously…YES! It was awful" I replied in total confusion.

"Not mine. I didn't feel a thang! I had him yesterday in the ambulance. He just slipped right out" she replied. As she exited the room, my mom said, "She must be on crack!"

Kevin was everything that everyone said he was. He was a beautiful baby with bright eyes, a button nose, cute little lips, and a head full of long curly hair. He was such a peaceful baby too. My parents' home was always filled with guests but with a new baby in the house it was more than normal. After six weeks, it was time to get back to school and I was ready. In the mornings, I had to wake up extra early and get both Kevin and myself dressed. It was school for me and the sitter for him. Every day my mom and I walked out the door with a baby, a book bag, a diaper bag, and purses. If we were ahead of schedule, she took me to the sitter's house first, then to school. But if we were running late, she would take me to school first, then take Kevin to the sitter.

On the days I sought *teenage* normalcy, I would catch the city bus with my friends. On those days, my mom would make a solo trip to take Kevin to the sitter. Due to my cosmetology program, my school days ran about 2 hours longer than the average student. After school each day, I was off to the sitter to pick up my little bambino.

Most nights after being in school all day I would have two to three hair clients. This was my way to get money so that I could cover daycare expenses, pampers, clothes etc. After finishing my client's services, I had homework. My mom and sisters were a big help. They assisted with bathing and sometimes feeding Kevin. It was like my dad said, 'We will care for him as a family!" The whole house pitched in to help. My mom deserved the "Trooper's Award". She took me to every doctor's appointment before, during and after the baby's birth. She also took me to school and picked me up every day.

My dad worked second shift. Yet, almost every day he brought home polish boys, wings and fries with sauce. It was no mystery how I gained 45 pounds while carrying a 7 lb. baby. Thank God I managed to leave the hospital 20 lbs. lighter than when I showed up.

Time was flying by. Kevin was now two years old. Together we all made it through my tenure in high school, my vocational course of cosmetology, and my freshmen year of college!

During this time, I didn't really pause much to look at my accomplishments. I had more goals than achievements and a child to raise. So, I was busy focused on what needed to be done next. My life was filled with Kevin, school, church and clients. Spiritually, I had become grounded. On Sunday mornings, we attended church faithfully. Every Wednesday I would fast to seek guidance and clarity for Kevin and I. I fasted the old school way, which means I substituted food with prayer, meditation and reading of the bible. On some Thursday nights, I even attend a praise service.

CHAPTER 2

THE WEEKEND

Friday July 19, 1997

I started my first stylist job at Abracadabra Hair and Nail Salon. Billy Dale, my uncle, owned the salon and he had a station waiting for me! My station was next to *Tomorrow Dawn*'s station, my cousin. The first day of work was great. The salon had great energy! To top it off, my clients had a more quality experience when coming to me for services.

Saturday morning, Mylon called and asked if he could get Kevin for the weekend, and of course I agreed. Free weekend for me!

Mylon and Kacie, were together. Although she and I had a tumultuous past, I never worried about Kevin being at their house. Kevin was always excited at the mere mention of going with his father. The only issue that I had was after Kevin would come home, he always smelled like Chinese food and bad cologne. For the life of me, I couldn't understand that. The smell drove me crazy. Immediately, I would throw him in the tub and his clothes in the washer.

This Saturday evening as we approached the white metal screen door, Kevin began to bang as if his life was in danger and he needed immediate access. "Kevin stop. That's rude. Trust me they can hear you." I tried to explain to him. The last thing I needed was for Mylon or Kacie to think that it was me beating on their door.

As soon as the door opened Kevin darted into the house like an arrow. He took off so fast, I still had his backpack in my hand. He was always excited to play with Mylon Jr. who like Kevin was two years old and his little brother

Karson, who was one years old. As Kacie stood in the doorway eyeballing me, I called out, "Kevin, come here,!" He came outside on the porch and I kneeled down so we could exchange hugs and kisses. Then, I opened his backpack and handed him a handful of freeze pops.

"Be sure to share with your brothers." I said.

"I will mommy!" He said with excitement.

"I Love you son." I replied.

"Love you mommy!" I responded back.

"I'll see you Monday." Were my last words to him.

I stood watch and laughed as he darted back into the house with his overstuffed backpack that was hanging from his little body. I headed back to the car. My friend Tamia and I had Beachwood Mall plans and later that evening I had a date. I hadn't been on one of those in about a year.

Rawls was bravado! He was the Blair Underwood type… beautiful dark skin, curly hair, long eye lashes, and a walk that oozed confidence. That evening at about 9pm, he picked me up in a van. Before I knew it the van was loaded with the two of us, and 3 of his male friends and their dates. We had a ball! The Flats of Downtown Cleveland was packed as usual. We all decided on pizza. On Lake Erie's banks, we ate and laughed the night away. All of the guys, except Rawl's best friend friend Will, had gone to Cleveland Heights High School too. So the table was full of "what have you been up to greetings" and high school memories." That night, the weather was perfect and so was the energy of everyone at our table.

As our server announced the restaurant was closing in five minutes, I looked at the time. It was 2:25 AM. I was 19 years old, but I still had a 2:30 AM curfew. I was hoping to be the first one dropped off since I was the first one picked up. However, my pride wouldn't allow me to utter my thoughts. I refused to humiliate myself by announcing that I was still on curfew. I was the third drop off. As we drove down my street at 3:15 AM, I could see that my father was standing on the porch. As we pulled up in front of the house, all I could think is, this is about to be really embarrassing. Then I realized it wasn't my father. It was my cousin Jeff! I was instantly relieved. With a smile, I said good night to everyone as I tried to exit the van swiftly. However, Rawls was a true gentleman and requested to walk me to the door. I quickly declined, as I urged *"No!"* No need. I'll be fine. My cousin is on the porch."

My dad is a night owl, and I couldn't take the chance of him coming to the door while Rawl's was walking me to the door after curfew.

As I walked up on the porch, Jeff was giving me the business. "It is very late, and I was worried about you."

I walked into the house and to my surprise, I found my sister Kisha, little sister Shelena, and our friend Tamia up watching a movie. My parents were asleep. Kisha informed me they went to bed hours ago. Thank goodness!

Sunday went as usual. I went to church that morning and that evening I went skating with my friend Tiffany Artist aka T.A.

Monday morning, I woke up with the biggest smile! I had just had a fantastic weekend!

CHAPTER 3

CAST DOWN

"Tina pick up the phone. It's Mylon," Mom yelled out from downstairs.

"Hello?" I said as I answered the phone.

"Hey Tina, I'm about to bring Kev home."

"Great! See you in a minute." I replied.

I'd had one incredible weekend, but I missed my son and I couldn't wait to see him. I looked at my clock and it was 9:17 am. I had just awakened, and there was no better way to top off my amazing weekend. Whenever Kevin and I were reunited, his eyes would light up, and he would run to me and scream "*Mommy!*"

I would pick him up in my arms, and we would share hugs, kisses and smiles! Picking him up from daycare was always a treat for me. That kid loved his momma, and I loved him back.

I rushed down stairs in preparation for his arrival. Mylon only lived 5 minutes away. With school being out for the summer and the salon being closed on Monday, I had planned for it to be our day! We would start off with breakfast, baths, and then off to the park.

While preparing his breakfast the phone rang. I looked at the caller ID, and I could see that it was Mylon. After I said hello, he proceeded "Tina, Jae is here and he's about to walk out the door. I'm not quite ready yet, but Kev is ready to come home now. He is crying because he wants to leave with him. Are you okay with Jae bringing Kevin home?"

"Sure that's fine!" I replied.

About 10 minutes later the phone rang, and the caller ID identified it to be Mylon again.

"Hello?"

"TINA!!! Jae just called! Kevin got hit by a car on Noble Road! I'm going up there right now!!" Mylon yelled.

Before I could let go of the receiver the phone rang yet again. Out of instinct I answered.

"Hello?" I could barely get the word out.

"May I speak with Tina?" I heard.

"This is her," I replied, "but I'm sorry I can't talk right now I have an emergency."

Then the voice on the line said, "Tina this is John Doe from Rainbow, Babies, and Children Hospital. Your son Kevin has been hit by a car. He's in the ambulance now..."

My dad overheard the conversation as I repeated some of what was being said. He rushed out the back door. I wanted to do the same, but I was still in my pajamas. After throwing on the first decent thing that I could find, my mom and I jumped in her car en route to the hospital. While riding, I got lost in my thoughts. I wondered if he would have a cast on his arm? Or maybe his leg? Or Both? However both seemed a bit extreme, so I figured I would just wait to get to the hospital to see what's going on.

But my mind didn't rest. I began to reminisce. The previous month, my church had a family day at Sea World. My Aunt Faleace and I, along with some of my cousins, had gone as a family. At some point after the dolphin show, we all ended up in the arcade. Kevin wanted to ride the motorcycle so I put him on one. Then I realized I didn't have any coins left, but if I had taken him off, another child would certainly take his spot. I asked my cousin Jon to watch him while I went for more coins. He said, "Sure." Two minutes later I came back to find Jon riding the motorcycle next to the one that Kevin was on.

"Jon, where's Kevin?" I asked.

"Ummm, he was just right here." Jon said while looking around to see if he

GLORY AND BLUES

could spot Kevin.

The search party was on. The whole family was now looking for him, and he was not within the four walls of the arcade. I stepped out of the arcade into masses of people. I could barely see in front of me. I had never been so scared and hopeless at the same time. My mind kept going back to a movie I'd seen many times as a child about an abducted little boy.

At some point, I stopped and looked up towards the sky. For a second everything around me ceased. The only thing that mattered was *my* direct *connection to God*. I uttered "Not like this. God please, help me. I can't leave this park without my child. I have to find him." I heard my name being called. I looked down and Tomorrow was standing in front of me with Kevin in her arms.

She said, "Girl, I found him sitting on a bench talking to some old people. This couple had to be eighty years old." They said that "they realized he was lost, but he didn't seem to know that he was lost. He just sat down and started talking about life." They decided they would listen and hopefully his parents would find him soon.

I looked back up towards the sky and said, "Thank you God." I realized *this was totally my fault*. My cousin was only 10, but I figured it would be okay. The change machine was only 30 feet away, and there was no line. I took Kevin in my arms and carried him to the car. It was certainly time to go.

There was another incident prior to that where Kevin was out in the yard with my parents. He was playing as they did yard work. I rushed outside. When I got out there, I found my father frantic as my mother stood holding Kevin while he hollered. "You're not going to believe what just happened. Kevin was playing with his toys while I was sweeping the sidewalk. The next thing I know I see a car flying down the street. Out of my peripheral, I see Kevin flying down the driveway on your brother's bike. It all happened so fast. I had to put the end of the broom stick in the spoke of the tire to stop him. Kevin flipped off the bike, but it was the only thing that stopped him from flying into the street." All I could say for the second time was, "Thank you God". I grabbed him in my arms. It was time to go back in the house. In that moment, I understood that I was the mother of a fearless little boy.

As we arrived to the hospital, my mom dropped me off at the door, and said "I'll park and you run in." Once I entered the lobby, I saw Kacie. Immediately, I remembered walking out of the skating rink the previous evening, and crossing the road to get to the parking lot where the car was parked. An oncoming car sped up as if it was trying to hit me. So I hurried across the street, only to look back and see Kacie as the driver. I had words for her, but this was not the time or the place.

I went over to the receptionist desk to ask which room Kevin was in. She overheard the receptionist as she was giving me directions, and Kacie said, "I know where the room is. I'll show you…"

Up the elevator we went. My mind kept picturing Kevin in a leg cast. We silently walked down the hall, and she showed me where the waiting room was. She entered the room first and immediately she sat on Mylon's lap. She began to caress his face with kisses while asking Mylon was he okay.

All I could think was she has to be the most immature, vexatious, repugnant person I know. If this was a show for me, she could really stop because I didn't want him. I was done with him the day I saw him at her locker.

I ignored her shenanigans and got to the point. "Mylon what happened?"

My dad burst into the room and repeated the question. "WHAT HAPPENED? How did Kevin get hit by a car?"

Mylon responded, "I don't know. He was with Jae and Kareem."

Mylon, Kacie, Kareem, my dad and I were the only ones in the room at that moment. So, I turned to Kareem and asked "What happened?"

He responded, "It's a long story."

Before I could get the words out of my mouth My dad yelled out, "A LONG STORY?? We got time!! What happened?" he asked again.

Kareem refused to say anything else as he just shook his head. Then my dad lost his composure and went off. All I can remember him saying is "My grandson just got hit by a car while with you and Jae, and all you have to say is it's a long story…?"

Kareem still stood there in silence. I was taken aback, speechless, and disgusted. I walked out of the waiting room. I saw Jae walking up the hall and met him halfway. As I approached him, his head hung low. I hugged him and then asked, "What happened?"

He said, "I decided to stop at the corner store before bringing Kevin home. I opened the car door and Kevin jumped out and started running. I called him. I even tried to catch him. It all happened so fast. The next thing I know is he was hit by a car." I simply replied "Okay."

After an hour the waiting room was filled with family, friends and some church members. The word had spread fast. The doctor finally entered the waiting room and he asked for the parents of Kevin. Before I got the chance to respond Kacie said, "We are his parents."

I walked up to the doctor and said "I AM Kevin's Mother!"

"He is Kevin's father" as I pointed toward Mylon, "and she is his father's girlfriend."

The doctor gave the report. "Kevin's neck is broken and his spinal cord is severely damaged. He is in a coma. He is brain dead, and he won't make it through the night." I couldn't believe what I had just heard and my faith could not conceive it either. As I stood face to face with the doctor, I asked him, "Has anyone ever recovered from such injuries?"

"No," replied the doctor.

"You are about to witness a miracle because Kevin will!" I persisted.

As the doctor walked out of the waiting room, it turned into an instant prayer zone. We were all praying and believing for a miracle. Shortly afterwards, the doctor announced that Kevin was ready for visitors. Of course, I was the first. I needed to be alone with him. The sight of my baby was unbelievable. My child was laid out on the hospital bed in a coma with a hard white brace around his neck. His physical body had minimum scars. Other than the neck brace, he looked fine. I reached to touch his hand, and his fingers were cold and so were his toes. Tubes were coming from every direction of his body. On top of his body was a baby blue heating blanket. Kevin was on life support. I was in disbelief as the tears ran uncontrollably down my face. But I tried to gather myself because I needed to be strong for him and for my family. I began to tell Kevin how he was going to be the hospital's miracle. I told him how much I loved and had missed him over the weekend.

Throughout that day we had so many visitors. Bishop Ellis was the only one who made me laugh. I was pleasantly surprised to see him. He arrived to the hospital shortly after my conversation with Jae. He said, in such a boisterous manner "I parked my car in front of the hospital doors and I dare somebody to tow me. I rushed up here as soon as your dad called me. I had to come and see about y'all!" His Presence was as loud and regal as it always was, but it was exactly what I needed at that moment.

The hours passed by as I watched my child fighting for his life. There were so many emotions that filled my heart: faith, fear, hurt, anxiety, and love. With every sound of the monitors, my heart would skip beats as fear rushed in. Truth is, I knew that God would come through. However, to watch my child lying helplessly was tough. As the day proceeded, the hospital had no shortage of people to come. By midday, confusion and anger began to set in. Different stories surfaced about how Kevin got hit by the car. Oddly enough, everyone said they got their story from the same person, Jae. I couldn't help but to think perhaps, is that was why Kareem declared it was a long story? Was there foul play involved? Had he chosen silence over a lie or the ugly truth?

Day eventually turned into night, and I was more than exhausted. Yet, I couldn't manage to close my eyes… not even for a second. My heart had been beating at such a rapid pace for twelve straight hours. My blood pressure had to be through the roof.

At midnight, while standing in the large waiting room that we had been transferred to due to the size of our crowd. My dad announced that he needed to take his mother (my Grandma Mary) home, and then he would head home as well for a little rest. He inquired about who was going to stay with me. Mylon was the first to speak up, "I'll be here."

Kacie quickly announced that she was staying too. I barely had any voice left, but mustered up enough to say "You can't stay." Then I looked at Mylon and said "she's gotta go."

My dad fully agreed and urged Mylon to escort her to her car. Mylon concurred and did just that.

I walked back to Kevin's room where my mom was standing by his bedside. I placed myself to the left side of the bed, and I began to whisper "I love you" in his ear. His fingers began to move and his eyes began to flutter. My mom said, "Whatever you just said to him he heard you and liked it!"

Within minutes the heart monitor screamed a boundless cry of fatality, one that I have never forgotten. The sound made my already rapidly beating heart race even faster. Suddenly, the doctor and nurses flooded the room. I could see what was happening, but stood there in disbelief. In the background I could even see and hear my mother screaming out "NO, not my Kevin!!"

I stood there in silence. I tried to rationalize it. This is not happening, I kept thinking.

This can't be real.

But it was happening. It was real.

Kevin passed away at 12:25am.

FOREVER CHANGED

He left and so did I.

I went into shock.

When I last saw him he was bubbling over with energy. And now, he was lifeless. *Where was my miracle*??... The one I'd been singing about in church since I was a little girl. Why had it evaded me?

As I stood at his bedside, the doctor looked at me and said "I am sorry but he is gone."

The pain was so intense I thought my heart would stop beating. In that moment, I wanted to die too. How could I live after such a tragic loss? I began to silently plead with God to please let me die. My heart went from beating like the speed of light to my body feeling totally numb. I could no longer feel my heart beating and I thought certainly this must be my end. After a few minutes there I still stood.

The range of emotions was so violent that I understood suicide. I embodied the hopelessness of the moment to come…Where the pain is so heightened that you can't see how it could ever take abeyance, let alone go away. A moment where it feels like the only way of escape is to no longer exist.

Side Bar: *I don't condone suicide—not then and certainly not now. I refused to conspire with the adversary regarding my life. It's impossible to no longer exist because we are eternal beings. To be absent from earth is to be present in a permanent reality; our souls live on forever. I couldn't bear to stand before my creator after destroying* *that which he created: my life. So, I silently begged God to please let me die.*

Like the walking dead, I was a zombie. In total anguish I exited the room. My heart had been *cast down into the deepest of hurts*. I turned down the hall as I walked a final jaunt from his room. I didn't know where I was going or what to do next. I could see that my body was moving, but I was so numb that I couldn't feel the ground underneath my feet. I was absent and present in one reality. Kevin was more than just my son. He was my reason and my conversation. He was the most beautiful part of me; *my heartbeat*. Now he was gone.

For 14 hours I had walked up and down these halls. This time as I made my way towards the waiting room, my Auntie Faleace looked upon me and she screamed, "NO!!" She must have seen death in my body. I nodded with a yes in confirmation. I was still surrounded by much family and friends, but I needed some time alone. I went straight into the private waiting room.

My first words were to my dad, who had just left the hospital. I paged him and he abruptly called back.

"Daddy, Kevin is gone.

He just died." I cried and in slow motion I dropped the phone.

Mylon rushed into the room.

"WHAT HAPPENED???" he asked.

"He's gone" I told him.

"But, I only walked away for five minutes to walk her to the car and just like that he's gone?" he asked in total confusion.

My eyes burned of fire. Throughout the day I had cried the ocean *blue*, but in this moment no tears fell.

We sat there on the sofa, empty.

Eventually, Mylon and I were escorted to a room and seated at an executive table with my parents, Grandma Prince, Mylon's mom Ms. Lacy, the doctor, and the coroner. Swiftly, they began to ask questions like, "Would you like to donate his organs to other children in need?"

I can remember being asked three times about donating his eyes but I can't remember if I said yes or no or if I answered the question at all. I was in no position to be asked anything, especially questions like this.

To all of our surprise, when they said "I'm sure Kevin didn't have life insurance," Ms. Lacy spoke up from across the table and said, "Yes he does. Kevin is insured! I have insurance on all my children and grandchildren."

To this day I am grateful for her. Kevin's funeral expenses were over nine thousand dollars.

That night I left the hospital *forever changed.*

CHAPTER

4

LIVE ON

In the spirit of moving forward, I told myself that God was giving me a *second chance*.

Over the next few days, funeral arrangements were made. Things that no parent should ever have to consider became my toil. What size, brand, and color coffin would you like? What kind of flowers would you like? Where would you like to lay him to rest? What will be his final outfit? Headstone?, etc. Each question shredded my heart even more.

The word of my son's death seemed to spread like dandelions. The doorbell and the phone rang nonstop. Every day, our house was full—as if it were a Fourth of July cookout. People brought buckets of chicken, mashed potatoes, biscuits, green beans, pies, and tons of other food. Most days we had more food than people. And every day we had tons of people.

On July 28, 1997, I woke up hoping that it was all a nightmare. But No. It was not. "This was really happening. Today was Kevin's funeral." From my bedroom I walked down the steps in an all-white suit. In the living room stood my parents, my grandparents, my siblings, Ms. Lacy, Mylon, his little brother and sister, and some additional family, everyone had been waiting on me.

As the limousines transported us to the church, I found myself staring out of the window while taking lots of deep breaths. I never saw trees so green, so defined, and so beautiful. At some point I lowered my eyes; to the left of us I saw both Tyra Henderson and Patrice Wilkerson, my old *tiger-nation* classmates. I looked around and realized our limousine was surrounded by cars with people that I knew. As we pulled into the parking lot of Pentecostal Church of Christ, people were standing outside. I thought maybe they were waiting on the family to enter first. But as we walked into this large sanctuary it was full. We were surrounded by family, friends, classmates, neighbors, my teachers, church members and Kevin's daycare teachers, his peers and their parents. I looked around and noticed all the pews, hallways and the balcony of the church was filled.

In my mind I replayed how every local news station had called but I declined all interviews. My name was never mentioned on the news only Kevin's. "How did everyone find out?" I wondered. All of these people were here to support me? To support Mylon? To support us? My eyes released a flood of tears.

A host of local bishops and pastors were in attendance, including the late Bishop Bill McKinney, Pastors Darrell and Belinda Scott. Many pastors, some that I didn't know came and gave their condolences. Pastor Belinda Scott, spoke such encouraging words, "With every loss there is a gain. *Look for the gain.* Tina, God is going to give you more than you anticipate".

As I viewed my child's lifeless body, I tried not to focus so much on the reality that my son was lying in that casket, but on the great job that his Grandma Lacy had done. Emotionally, I could not shop for my son's last outfit. So she offered to do it for me. He was dressed in an all-white suit. After I got back to my seat, sorrow consumed me.

During the memorial viewing, people would come by and love on me. I received tons of hugs, kisses, flowers and cards. A man walked up to me. He was so close to my face our noses almost touched. "I am so sorry about your loss. I am praying for you" he said. This man was the most unattractive man I had ever seen. As he walked away, I looked over to my mom who sat to my immediate right and I asked, "W H O was that?" Maybe it was my facial expression or the length of the "*WHO*" in my statement…or both. I don't know… but she looked at me and tried to answer but only laugher came out. Before we knew it, we were bent over in uncontrollable laughter. The more we tried to stop, the funnier it became. Once again tears flooded our faces but this time it was different. We received a momentary escape from the solemnity of the ceremony. That laughter provided me with the strength that I needed to continue in that service.

Pastor Gwen McCurry, continued the service with prayer. "God impart strength, peace, joy and minister love to these parents and to this family". She proclaimed "Using praise during testing times helps to make smooth transitions".

Scriptures were read by children from Pentecostal Church of Christ, Christopher Williams and David Cunningham read: scriptures Isaiah 57:1 and John 14:1-4.

Solos were sang by Sharon Clark and Kevin Frazier

Bishop Jesse D. Ellis, was the next to address the congregation. With such clemency he conveyed "I don't understand *WHY* this was allowed to happen... But what I do know is...

- God has something to say. We're just not ready to hear it yet.
- God has an explanation for why this was permitted.
- God will get around to explaining this, either now or later. There won't be any question left unanswered.
- We don't always understand God, yet we trust him.

Bishop then read the obituary. When he got to the part which he had personally written, it brought a smile to my face:

> *At such a young age, we have no way of knowing whether or not Kevin really understood all the message of Christ, but we do know that he loved and was loved by the Lord and his family. "Have you ever watched Kevin dance before the Lord?"*
>
> **We did!**
>
> *On Sunday before last, Kevin joined the saints in praise and while acting like the saints, he ran into the drums. Grandpa Lindsey picked him up and brought him back to his pew. Then in a moment or so, Kevin was at it again!*
>
> *Kevin began his eternal dance and praise on July 22, 1997. "Good-bye" here is just "good morning" over there. If we would live as Christ would have us to live, we will see Jesus when our time comes to die. There will be another bonus for those who knew Kevin. We'll see him again.* **What a reunion!**

I wasn't there that Sunday. I didn't even know that he had gotten *his shout* on at church. He certainly wasn't a shy kid, so it didn't shock me. Whenever I played music at home, we would dance together. When I played gospel, Kevin would cut a rug!

Elder Michelle Williams, *(now Pastor Michelle Moore)* sang "I WILL MAKE THE DARKNESS LIGHT". I'm sure all of heaven stood still as her pipes powerfully executed that *hymn*.

THEIR SCAR

Bishop Eric Clark preached a sermon entitled "THE POWER OF DEATH".

He highlighted the scripture, "*To every thing there is a season, and a time to every purpose under the heaven: A time to be born, and a time to die,* - Ecclesiastes 3:1-2"

His message was bold, spell-binding and radical!

"*Death can do what a lot of things cannot do...*

- Death can bring families together that haven't been together in years.
- Death can make iron-men cry.
- Death can cause the denominational divide to unite: bishops, pastors, reverends, and ministers that won't normally come together, will come together for death.
- Death caused Abraham to show his true faith in God.
- Death caused Rizpah to watch guard over her son's dead bodies for 7 months.
- Death can cleanse and give the whole world another chance.

Jesus taught, prayed and walked on water, he open blinded eyes, he healed the sick and raised the dead, but that didn't bring man back to God. God used his secret weapon called Death.

Jesus died until the sun wouldn't shine. Jesus died until the moon cried blood. Jesus died until earth began to quake. Jesus died until the soldier said "Surely this is the son of God". God took his own son's life, so that we could be saved.

GLORY AND BLUES

Tina, what if God took your son's life to save a soul, would that be a good enough reason?"

Bishop Clark, followed his sermon with an Alter Call. "Could it be that you're here today and Kevin died for you? To get your attention… Today we are here for Baby Kevin. Tomorrow it could be you… "Is your life is order?"

Side Bar: *I have been to a lot funerals and I never seen or heard of an outpour like this. The alter was flooded with no less than 100 people. There was an intense cry of worship, repentance and surrender.*

After the alter call Bishop Clark prayed. "Let the day come, that they (Kevin's parents) can show *their scar* and stand up and say, [*"this is my scar"*]. This is what the Lord did *in me*. Someday the *pain, frustration* and *confusion will aid others* through their pain, frustration, and confusion. Lord, we accept that your taking of young Kevin is just another way that you are using this family".

Towards the end of the service, Bishop Ellis called Mylon and I, up to the altar. As we faced the crowd of people, he led the congregation in prayer for us. While he prayed, I held Mylon's hand. We hadn't been together since the day we conceived Kevin and I knew we'd never be together again. But in that moment… for a second time we stood in unity at this altar. The first time was when Bishop Ellis prayed blessings over our new born son.

At the end of the funeral service before we headed to the cemetery, I saw Rawls and his best friend Will. I couldn't believe he was there. I went over to them and gave them a hug. I also thanked them for coming out.

I couldn't help but to ask, "I thought your boss wouldn't let you off?"

"He didn't. I got fired, but this is far more important." He replied.

After the funeral was the repast. After the repast, our home was once again jammed packed…for several days actually. People came from everywhere to love on us. We would all watch movies, laugh, cry, eat, play cards, Boggle, etc. Every night, my cousin Andre managed to find himself in the kitchen washing dishes.

Side Bar: *There is a major misconception that the funeral is the toughest part of death. Reality is, prior to the funeral you're busy planning and entertaining guests. The conclusion of the funeral is when living out the reality begins.*

LIFE AFTER DEATH

Every morning bright and early, I woke up to three phone calls. The first call came from Bishop Ellis with "TINA - How are ya? What are you doing today? The Lord loves ya Girl!" One day he called me later than usual. "Well, Tina I'm calling you a little late today. We are at Disney World on vacation. The girls wanted to release balloons to Heaven, so today we did." I believe the Lord was gracious enough to give Kevin his balloons!

The second call came from Rawls. He had landed another job and on his way to work, he would call me. If he was able to determine that I was okay, then he would go on to work. However, he would detour to my home if he could tell that I had been crying. It didn't matter to him what his boss thought. He said he could get another job, but my well-being was top priority.

The third call came from Tomorrow with how are you doing? What are you doing today? And I love you.

It had been 2 weeks since Kevin's passing. Life didn't stop because I was experiencing a tragedy. No, it kept going and so did I. *Emotional Intelligence* became my resolve. I was afraid to slow down. I felt that too much idol time with *pain this intense* could lead to danger: drugs, alcohol or *something destructive*. So, I didn't touch any of it. Any substance would have become an addiction. I needed relief, but the kind that ONLY God could provide.

One morning, I stood in the mirror and told myself, "I can't change what happened to me on yesterday, but today *I won't be life's victim*." Moving forward and putting it all behind me seemed like mission impossible. Every day I missed my baby more than the day before. "I wanted my son back!" My anger with Jae, Kareem, Mylon, and God constantly grew. I was angry with Jae for having inconsistencies in his story and I constantly wondered what really happened that day, with Kareem for choosing silence in the mist of tragedy, Mylon for remaining friends with Kareem and Jae, and God for allowing this to happen.

On the third week, I returned back to work, and Rawls and I had our second date. It was really like a first date because it was just the two of us. We went out to dinner but only after he took me to his home to meet his parents. They were so warm and kind towards me. As we were leaving for dinner, they walked us outside. Rawls opened my car door as his parents stood on the sidelines giving high-fives as Mr. Aldoson affectionately held his Mrs. in his arms. His parents quickly grew to love me, and I loved them too. It seemed as if I spent more time at their house than at my own. The highlight of my day became Rawls pulling up in the driveway. I always felt rescued. His gold Diamante was as dope as the vibe inside of his car. He would bump Sade, 112, Biggie, Erykah Badu, Lauren Hill or Wu Tang. Within minutes, I was out of my reality and infused into his. It was better than Calgon, as he would take me away.

At our home guests eventually stopped coming and calling because I stopped being there. I couldn't handle being home anymore. Everything in the house made me think about Kevin, especially my little brother and his pictures of Kevin proved to be more than I could handle.

My brother Derval was born with the umbilical cord around his neck. I wasn't there, but I was told he was rushed out of the delivery room. His development was delayed due to his struggle at birth, and he never developed language skills. His cognitive development was such that he could not grasp sign language either. But Derval and Kevin loved one another. By the time Kevin was one year old he was probably the only real friend that Derval had. Mom used to say being in the house with the two of them was like being in the house with Tom and Jerry. You would never hear words only sounds as they fussed and wrestled.

At 10 years of age, Derval tried to be as gentle as he could with Kevin because he understood that he was much bigger than him. Kevin was rough, though. Perhaps it was just his nature, but Kevin and I would watch WWF often. I was addicted to watching wrestling. I lived for the moment "Can you smell what the Rock is cooking?" For me it was only entertainment. It was a different story for Kevin. He was studying moves that he could practice on Derval. When Derval was tired and had had enough of Kevin jumping on his neck and pounding on him, he would pick Kevin up and put him in his playpen. Soon Kevin learned how to climb out of it, and it was like being in the cartoon with the famous cat and mouse. We couldn't seem to get either one of them to stop wrestling or fussing. Yes, it was crazy but that was the Lindsey's household! I was glad that Derval finally had a playmate. Kevin was someone who didn't make fun of him, but loved him unconditionally. Together they did what boys do.

Before the funeral, my mom and I tried to explain to Derval that Kevin was gone and never coming back. We even tried to explain at the cemetery. If I asked Derval to bring me the phone, he would. If I said give this to mommy for me, he would. If I asked him if he was hungry, he would say "yeah" or shake his head no. Yet, I don't know if he understood this, that Kevin was dead and never coming back. I could barely wrap my mind around it. My parents are both photographers so our home was loaded with pictures. Everyday Derval would bring me a picture of Kevin. He was communicating very clearly. He wanted Kevin, [his Jerry] back, and so did I.

WHY?

Many days, I pondered why this was happening to me. It's like repeating a nightmare. Surreal. Unfathomable. I didn't just lose my son that day. *I lost emotional freedom.* I lost the ability to feel normal. I lost faith in "God will come through" and it was replaced with the belief that "God will come through *"IF"* he chooses to." The longing, hurt, disappointment, and confusion were very real and controlled my every thought. I could not think about Kevin without totally breaking down. He was MY CHILD. Age had no barrier on my ability to love my son. I could not understand how God would allow this to happen to me. The most sensitive girl in the world…that was me as a growing up. I would cry at the drop of a dime. As a teenager, I learned to better control my emotions but I was still that girl and this was so far beyond anything that I could handle. I was only nineteen years old. In three years, I had gone from being a regular everyday teenager to a mom with responsibilities, then to the death of my son.

Theoretically, I just couldn't comprehend this; my relationship with God wasn't new. We had a history and I trusted him. HOW could he love me and allow this to happen? I didn't give into the notion "that I must have done something wrong…" That's Karma and God doesn't function in that way. But the question still remained… *WHY?*

TARRYING ROOM

As a little girl, my family and I were members of Christ Temple Apostolic Church. The Sunday's that I didn't volunteer in the nursery, I would sit in the sanctuary and listen to each word as the choir sang. I found myself singing along to those songs at church and at home. Bishop Halton would preach and most times I would fall asleep. I always woke up during alter call. I was fascinated with the idea of having a relationship with God. At 8 years old, I got saved. I can still remember walking down the aisle to the altar saying "I want to be saved." It was a simple process, I just had to *B.R.A.C.E* myself; Believe, Repent, Accept, Confess and Endure. Shortly after getting saved, I got baptized. Then I decided I wanted more meaning I wanted that Holy Ghost too. One Sunday, during the alter call when the invitation got to the part of "Does anyone want to tarry for the Holy Ghost?" I escorted myself down the aisle again. I was already a member. I was already saved and I had been baptized. I just needed to finalize the work.

I was escorted to the basement by one of the elder church mothers. The church basement wasn't a new scene for me. That's where the restrooms, the nursery and Sunday School for children was held. But the *tarrying room* was new to me.

The church mother began to explain that "the Holy Ghost is a gift from God. If you really want it with all of your heart, then God will give it to you with the evidence of speaking in tongues." So go ahead and start calling on the name of Jesus. And so I did: "Jesus, Jesus, Jesus, Jesus, Jesus, Jesus… Jesus, Jesus, Jesus, Jesus, Jesus, Jesus. Jesus, Jesus, Jesus, Jesus, Jesus, Jesus, Jesus…"

After about an hour, I was *tongue twisted* and *tired* with a runny nose! The elder mother said "It's okay baby," and patted me on the back. "You didn't get it today." I was as sad as could be. I wanted that *"keeping power"* that Bishop Halton and Grandma Prince was always talking about. After weeks of failed attempts, one day while at home I was reading my bible and I began to pray. "Lord, I want the Holy Ghost. The bible says it is a gift to those who ask for it, and I am asking for it. Lord please fill me with the Holy Ghost."

The next Sunday I stayed awake for the entire service. I found myself standing before the pastor during altar call. Bishop Halton smiled at me and said somebody take little Lindsey down to the tarrying room. This time it was two church mothers. I had memorized their spiel so I got straight on my knees and started calling on the name of Jesus. "Jesus, Jesus, Jesus, Jesus, Jesus." At the sixth Jesus, I heard such a calm and peaceful voice "COME UNTO ME THIS DAY MY CHILD." Immediately I began speaking in tongues. I could hear the older church mothers saying [*"She got it*!] This time she got it!!!" It flowed like the river. The spirit of God was all over me. I got up off of my knees. I began to shout aka (also known as) dance while speaking in tongues. I had no idea what I was saying, but I felt amazing. When I finally opened my eyes, I noticed my grandmother and mother were shouting along side of me and speaking in tongues too. At eight years of age, *I got that keeping power*!

As a teenager, I found out that keeping power doesn't stop you from doing wrong. Instead, it puts conviction deep down in your heart, which makes wrong "*doing*" as uncomfortable as a pair of too tight shoes. By no stretch of the imagination has my spiritual walk been perfect. I am flawed and I've had my fair share of mishaps. Some of them I enjoyed and some I didn't. Nonetheless, I always returned unto the Lord with a heart of repentance.

I know my heavenly father, my relationship with Him is real and no his ways aren't new to me, but I still couldn't understand, *WHY ME?*

I was left feeling betrayed. He closed his eyes and allowed my child to be hit by a car and then allowed him to die.

At night, I would cry myself to sleep. Upon awaking before I could even open my eyes they were filled with tears and I would weep. I was shattered, beyond measure.

Spiritually I found myself in an awkward space. I was *mad as hell* with God, but I knew that I needed Him. My anger caused a disconnect, and I struggled communing with Him, but my soul would sing *hymns* and worship songs like the ones I learned as that little girl.

I SURRENDER ALL
All to Jesus I surrender;
All to Him I freely give;
I will ever love and trust Him,
In His presence daily live.

I surrender all, I surrender all;
All to Thee, my blessed Savior,
I surrender all.

CHAPTER

5

EXERTION

God knew what was to come. He even sent me a few signs. Instead of preventing the accident, he allowed it. The *first sign* was the disappearance at the park. The *second sign* was that day with the bike episode. I walked into the bathroom to brush my teeth. As I looked in the mirror I didn't see me. I saw a vision, and it was my child on a bike. He was flying down the driveway and a car was coming. I called on Jesus, and just like that the vision went away. I wiped the tears from my face, then I brushed my teeth, and proceeded outside. As I got to the front door I could hear Kevin hollering. I rushed outside and my father informed me of what had just happened with Kevin, but I didn't tell my parents about the vision I had experienced. How could I? I didn't quite understand how that was possible. The *third sign* was during my freshman year of college. My friend Dion would pick me and my friend named Keisha up for school. He lived around the corner from us. One morning Keisha stayed home... so while Dion and I were riding to school he began to tell me how he couldn't sleep at all the night before.

"I was up crying all night," he said.

"Why?" I asked him.

"I don't know why." He replied.

I didn't have any advice to offer so I just listened. After my first class, I spotted him in the cafeteria.

"Hey! You okay?" I asked.

He couldn't answer because *his eyes were fixated* on a man in an all-black suit

A BOLD PERSPECTIVE

with a white clergy collar who had just entered the cafeteria.

As the man passed us, Dion said, "Excuse me sir. I don't mean to bother you, but would you have bible study with me?"

The man looked very confused. He replied, "I can't even remember WHY I came up here so sure, I'll have bible study with you."

Dion and the man took a seat at an available table. I joined them along with another girl from my English class. The man opened his bible and read a short passage of scripture, and then said, "Let's pray." As he was calmly praying, the girl began to say. "Hallelujah! Thank you Jesus." She wasn't loud, but it was enough for me to give her a side eye.

He ended his prayer, and to my surprise he raised his head and said to her, "You have a big mouth and you need to learn how to shut up. Nobody likes you. The one person who is kind to you, you mistreat."

I was stunned. I realized we were convening with a real prophet. The bible clearly states that prophets are those who God speaks through. I'd seen people be mean to her and cause her shame and embarrassment. She struggled with low self-esteem. While in class the day before, she was so nasty towards me. I chose to let it go, because I felt sorry for her. The last thing that she needed was for me to treat her the way others treated her or how she was behaving towards me. The prophet proceeded to tell her more personal things about her life as she wept.

Next, he looked at Dion and said, "So, you were up all night crying, huh?"

Dion's mouth fell open and his eyes were as big as quarters! He told Dion *why* he was crying and shared a host of other things with him.

He looked at me and I was ready as I had hoped for a word of *divine prosperity!*

"YOU." He said to me.

"*Put both your hands out with your palms up...*"

After *all* that he had spoken to me, I was left like Dion with my mouth wide open. The last thing he said to me was "get to class… you're late."

I looked up at the clock. I was indeed late…15 minutes late to be exact.

So again, God knew what was to come.

The summer had been emotionally grueling. By August, the return of the

GLORY AND BLUES

fall semester I had 21 credit hours, I worked part-time job at a salon, and part-time job at MBNA, a telemarketing company. Rawl's and I were still dating. I continued to skate every Sunday. Eventually, I even started skating on Thursday nights too. At all times I kept myself absolutely busy with something. Idle time became painful because it caused me to think about my reality. Whenever I felt a void, I would fill it with shopping, television or a telephone call with Tomorrow. I still attended church every Sunday. I needed the praise and worship. It would minister life to my broken heart. When the praise teams would sing GOD NEVER FAILS, I would hurt even more. My life was excluded from the grace of those words.

By the first anniversary of *the* death, I realized my life was full of people and stuff. Yet I was so empty. Nothing fulfilled me. One late night Rawls walked me to my door as he always did. I told him I couldn't do us anymore.

"What do you mean?" He asked.

"This relationship" I replied.

"I am emotionally, mentally and spiritually wreck. I love you, but spiritually I am so far gone, and I need God to heal me. He can't until I make space in my life.

He looked crushed; I couldn't look in his eyes another moment.

I said good-bye, and walked in the house. Through the peephole on the door, I watched him stand there for a several seconds. Then he turned away.

He called me a few days later, and boy was I happy to see his number on the caller ID. Everyday I wanted to call him, but I denied myself. Moments into our conversation, I was saddened as he reported that he was moving to New York.

"When?" I asked.

"Next week." he replied.

He was moving on with his life and I felt desolated. Life was happening to me, but it didn't seem to have my best interest. They say *"life is what you make it."* I say" *NOT always true."* I was in a real crisis. I had lost my son and now the best boyfriend I had ever had was moving away. I didn't mean for this to happen, I just needed some time to gather myself.

On his last day in the city, he invited me over. We had dinner with his parents, and I helped him pack a few last things. As his parents drove him to the bus station, I went along for the ride. The ride back was somber as I fought back the tears. I couldn't allow his parents to see me cry, so I shifted my thoughts.

"The reality was we were both 20 years old, and what we had was real. In the right timing, we'll pick back up where we had left off." At least, that's what I hoped for, or maybe it's just what I told myself so that I could move on. In the beginning, we talked almost every day. Once I even took a trip to New York to visit him. But after a few months we both stopped calling.

A year and a half had gone by and my world evolved. I finished junior college. I had my Associates of Liberal Arts. My original goal was to finish at Cleveland State with a bachelor's in business, but with Kevin gone and so was my motivation. I wasn't in school for me. It was for him. After his death, every class was grueling but I toughed it out.

Work was fun! My salon clientele was booming. I loved my clients and my co-workers. It was the highlight of my day. We worked long hours on Thursdays and Fridays. Sometimes, I didn't leave the salon until midnight. My co-workers, Tammy and Delisha, would work until 2 am sometimes. I thought they were crazy for that, but we were in our early twenties.

At church, I was on the adult dance ministry and assisted with the children's dance ministry. I was asked to head up the new member's ministry, so I did. I was also in training to be Pastor Lynora's (our pastor's wife) armor bearer (assistant). I was a busy church worker and I didn't mind. I had tons of time and no real responsibility.

Oh yeah, I managed to move on after Rawls. I began dating a young man that was a member and a leader in my church. He was the Minister of Music. He and I became pretty serious. He asked me to marry him and I agreed. A year earlier, I couldn't even imagine dating someone else, let alone being engaged! Flowers were delivered to my job regularly, sometimes he even hand delivered them, accompanied with lunch. He was very charming and fun. My life felt as if it was coming together and I was happy.

After a few months of being engaged, I realized there could be no marriage. He was out in the city sowing his royal oats. Emotionally, I had enough problems. I was still in mourning and the last thing I needed was a cheating husband. I had a couple of clients who had that problem. They all had the same side effect, a big bald spot in the center on their heads. They *all* said it was from stress. Well…that type of stress? I certainly didn't need in my life. No thank you Sir. I'm good. Goodbye!

During our engagement the thought of being married and having a new baby seemed to be the antidote for my sorrows. That was the hardest part of our breakup. My healing was in the palm of my hands and now I felt more wounded and disappointed than I was a year ago.

So naturally, I found myself thinking about Rawls. I had never really stopped thinking about him, but now he was heavy on my mind, so I called him.

"Yo! What's up Tina!! It's been a while!" He said.

"Yes it has been, Rawls," I replied.

I was all smiles while talking to him… then I had a Jill Scott moment.

"You're getting married??"

I tried not to give any indication of my real feelings, but I was deflated down to nothing as I listened to him share his good news.

I thought to myself, I had pushed away the best guy I would probably ever have.

CHAPTER 6

ALTERATION

One day on my way to work, which was only about six miles and three turns away from home, I could not remember how to get to the salon. I grew up on these streets and I had driven this same path for a couple of years now. But, I just could not remember the route. I pulled over in the Cedar Warrensville shopping plaza and had an emotional breakdown. In that moment, I realized I was losing my sanity. I cried out, "God help me because I am losing my mind." I stayed parked for a while and cried. Eventually I remembered the route and proceeded to work.

Free from most of my prior obligation, but still drowning in pain I knew that it was time for me to totally turn my focus to God! I hadn't missed a Sunday morning service since Kevin had passed and I had recently started attending Wednesday night service. But I knew a spiritually intimate relationship with God is far beyond showing up for service. The foundation of the relationship is communication and trust but my spiritual communication and trust had become extinct. My new philosophy was *"what will be…will be…"* so, what's the point of praying, trusting, and believing?

As I tried to navigate through this life that was coerced upon me Sunday service would give me the strength to make it to Wednesday then Wednesday back to Sunday! I wish I could say that after three years I found peace, but I didn't. I was grievously vexed. I had become a church addict and a shopping addict. If I was having a bad day or if I *thought* the day may take a sad turn… off to the mall I went. It was my comfort zone! At the mall, I would start with a pretzel and lemonade. I work my way to all my favorite stores! I never left the mall without bags.

In some ways life was getting better and I found myself getting stronger. I still loved my job and my co-workers. At church I did more praising then crying and I began to pray a little more. After Kevin's death spiritually I had lost trust, but I decided to trust God again with my *total life*. A few days after *that decision* my co-worker Delisha and I got tattoos. On my back I have a small cross with mandarin letters that say "*Trust God*". It is my outward symbol for my inward transformation. But even after this mental shift, I realized I still needed something else because I was still hurting *so much*. Shopping and church proved to only temporarily fill the void.

I needed more and it had to be very different.

One day while at work Delisha asked me to go to Atlanta with her for a hair show. So I did! It was my first time going to Atlanta and I loved it! Over the next two years I traveled to Atlanta six times. After my second visit, I started to consider Atlanta for my new place of residence. While in the city I felt an overwhelming sense of peace and calm. Atlanta was clean with bright sunshine. My spirit was awakened and I found myself open to new possibilities.

It was now eight years after my son's death. While packing and finalizing things for my move, my mom cleared out several of my drawers. She looked at me with concern and gently said "Okay… this bag is equivalent to a large garbage bag and it is filled to the top with just underclothes! I have never seen or heard of anyone with this many pair!" Though gentle in her approach, it was a stern reminder of how I had been living. *Grief Stricken*. The sad part is that bag of undergarments only represented a *very small* percentage of clothes I had accumulated in my efforts at therapeutic resolve. My shopping impulses gave a whole new meaning to the old adage of "*Retail Therapy*".

MARCH 2005

Relocation allowed me to reset! At the top of 2005, I had finally arrived to Atlanta. I brought with me my new GA licenses for cosmetology and real estate. (I had applied for the both of them a few months earlier). A big rented Penske Truck, which was filled with all of my retail therapy and my bedroom set. Let me clarify, little ole me didn't drive that truck. My dad drove the truck while my mom rode shotgun. Me? Well, I rode in the back seat of my car with two pillows and a blanket and with my feet propped up, while my cousin Andre and my friend Bryant drove my car. Driving Ms. Tina became the mission!

After arriving to my new apartment we all lugged what felt like hundreds of boxes that were filled with clothes and shoes up the stairs to my second floor apartment. The guys of course carried and assembled my bedroom set. After a very long day Andre' went home which was in Villa Rica just 30 minutes away.

After a day or so, my mom, dad and Bryant got me situated and then they flew back to Ohio. As I took them to the airport it was bitter sweet. I knew that I would miss not just them but everyone.

The night prior to the move I couldn't sleep. I began to think about everyone and everything that I would miss, my family, my church, my colleagues, my clients, my kill it skillet moments at Yours Truly with my best friend Marquetta, and shopping and dining-out play dates with Tomorrow. I would also miss Sunday night skating and going to the Cavs games, Lebron was on fire.

At 3am I stood in the restroom mirror trembling, while tussling back and forth with *fear -vs- courage*. I had almost changed my mind about moving to Atlanta. Then I focused in on a few realities. The truck was in the driveway fully loaded and my cousin Andre was asleep down stairs. He had flown from Atlanta to help with the drive. My car was his transport back home to his wife, Shandra and their children Stephanie and Danielle.

I then thought about Bryant and how much I would miss hanging out with him. He was a breath of fresh air! I met him maybe six months earlier. Tomorrow and I were out to Bahama Breeze. While finishing our dinner a guy came over to our table.

"Hey Ladies! Whuz up?"

"I'm Cortney."

"What's y'all names?" He said."

He was a little rough around the edges. He continued, "My uncle over there is a little shy."

I took a deep breath as I thought to myself, wait are they playing *shy guy*?

Cortney continued, "He wants to pay y'all bill."

I slowly looked backed expecting some old man, but he was maybe 32 years

A BOLD PERSPECTIVE

old. His uncle was a tall chocolate teddy bear with a great smile. Once the server came over to our table to deliver our bill, his uncle casually walked over and smoothly took the bill. Right away, he recognized Tomorrow. Her back had been turned to him the entire time. It turned out that they were from the same neighborhood, Miles. Bryant was the same age as her older brother, Jamal. After a great conversation, he asked me for my phone number. I was hesitant, but after conversing for quite a while I eventually gave it to him. I decided that if he was a bugaboo I would do as I had just done, change my phone number.

A few days later he called me. Oddly enough, life found us in the same space. I was not looking to be in a relationship and neither was he.

We both had a story. Mine was Kevin... Bryant was a single dad raising two daughters. Their mom who was the love of his life, she had been murdered. We didn't talk much about our hurts but as a result of what we had been through (losing a person very dear to us) we shared a respect for life and for one another's strive, to not just exist but to *LIVE (in spite of)*.

Bryant was a very thoughtful man and his laugh was like silk. I began to look forward to his calls. He was different from the guys that I knew. He worked for the city and he read the newspaper everyday. I was used to seeing older men read the paper, not young men. My dad didn't even read the newspaper. He only watched the news on television. Daily Bryant filled me in on the latest news because I didn't read the paper or watch the news. The first couple times he asked me out not as a date but as friend, I declined. I had just wrapped up a very weird situation that had me uninterested in going out.

About the weird situation… a month prior there was a guy who I had known for a year. We went to church together. He had asked me out once and I declined. He seemed like a very nice guy but he wasn't my type. A few months had gone by and he asked me out again. This time I said okay. Since my split with the musician two years ago I had been on a couple dates with guys that were my type and none of those guys worked out, so I decided *why not try something different.*

Our first date was great! It was my first five star experience. I was used to Cheesecake Factory, Olive Garden, Outback, J. Alexander, etc… Occasionally I would even eat at Applebee's. This boutique style restaurant was a very quaint. The atmosphere and the service was *amazing*.

GLORY AND BLUES

That night I ordered duck, asparagus and whipped potatoes. Over dinner we had a great conversation, but I didn't care much for my food. The asparagus was the weirdest veggie I had ever had, the duck carried a stench but the potatoes were delicious! After dinner he took me back home. He escorted me to my front door as he said, "I had a great time and I hope that we can do this again." I answered the invitation with "Thank you for such a great evening. Yes we can do this again!"

Our second date was just as nice. On our third date, while having dinner he said some things to me that I liked! "You are beautiful! I would love to spend the next 21 days showering you with *gifts. Gifts that either remind me of you, or gifts that I think that you would like.*" I melted into my chair. As I thought "HE might become my new type! A girl *like me* can get used to all of this." I only responded with a slight blush followed by "Wow! That sounds wonderful." Then mentally I left. I *perused* my grey matter like a file cabinet, but I came up short. I couldn't pinpoint one *chick flick* that had that line. Trust me, I have seen all the good ones and some bad ones too.

TWENTY-ONE DAYS

Day One: Which was the next day. I got a call from him saying, "Hey! Check your mailbox."

In the box, there was a disc titled "All Things Beautiful." The instructions read "place me in your hard drive." I did as instructed. It was a slide show with breathe taking images of mountains, oceans, flowers, pyramids, sunsets etc... At the end of the show there was a picture of me with creative font that spelled out "You Are Beautiful!"

I was flattered! It was a simple yet beautiful gesture. Might I add he drove 30 minutes each way to hand deliver a disc to my mail box.

Day Two: We met at a pizzeria. Upon my arrival he gave me a gift bag. It had several pairs of colorful socks. I love pizza and socks. *He was two for two!*

Day Three: I had a late morning flight to Atlanta and he wanted me to have my gift before I left town. That morning he came to my parent's house and handed me another gift, I was so excited! After I removed the tissue paper and all the contents from the gift bag me, my dad, and my 6 year old nephew, we all just looked. Shaun was the first to speak "OOH PLAY-Doh! Is that for me?"

He bought me Play-Doh, two changes of Barbie doll clothes and a fashion magazine. I was okay with the magazine; at that time fashion and shopping were my twist. The Play-Doh confused me and the Barbie clothes took me back to my childhood. I was never into dolls, so right away my mom stopped buying them for me. There I was disappearing into my grey matter once again. I kept thinking, *"What does he expect me to do with these toys?"* I have to believe the look on my face prompted him to quickly explain. "You are super creative and very fashion forward..." Everything else that he said next sounded like "blah, blah, blah." My dad was the next to speak as he said "Tina if you want to make your flight we need to leave now." I told Landon thank you and escorted him to the door.

As soon as he walked out I gave Shaun the Play-Doh. As my dad and I walked to the car he started laughing and I knew why. I joined in the laugher, but we didn't discuss it. There was nothing to say.

The previous month I had moved back home with my parents. I was relocating to Atlanta in six months, and staying with them would allow me to save my rent money as additional cushion for my move.

My weekend trip to Atlanta was both business and pleasure. After three days it was time to fly back to Cleveland. That morning Landon asked me if he could pick me up from the airport. He wanted to talk over dinner. I accepted. He was really a nice guy, but clearly he was missing something and so was I. On the way to the restaurant we discussed my trip.

"Did you find the area that you want to live in? How about a place to work?" He asked.

I answered, "I didn't find where I want to live or work, but I have crossed a few places off the list. I know where I don't want to live or work.

After entering the restaurant and confirming the reservations, the host escorted us to our table. Within minutes, our server arrived with an arrangement of flowers. "Courtesy of the gentleman" she said and then she walked away.

That was certainly a surprised. I had never had that happen before. He didn't just show up, he had thought this out ahead of time.

The server returned and asked, "Are you guys ready to order?"

I gave a quick, "yes," because I was starving. "I'll have the filet mignon, whipped potatoes and a salad. Ma'am it comes with two center pieces. How would you like them prepared?" she asked.

"Well done, please." I said.

"NO. Make hers medium." Landon replied.

I turned to him and said, "No, I don't like medium." Then, I turned back to the server and said, "Ma'am I'll have it well done please."

He spoke out again, "NO she'll have it medium."

At this point I was done trying to explain to him that I don't like mine prepared that way. I just stared at him.

After a few seconds I turned back to our server, and apologized. "Ma'am I am sorry. Please forgive us for the confusion. He will not be eating my meal... I'll have mines well done, please and thank you."

As she was taking his order, I couldn't believe what had just happened.

A. How Embarrassing.

B. How Controlling.

"Thank you I'll take the menus," the server said.

I patiently waited for her to leave the table, then I got straight to it. "WHY would you do that? That was so embarrassing."

"But, Tina the way you ordered your steak, it would be dry and tough. I want you to be able to enjoy your meal," he said,

I replied, "That's all fine and dandy for you, but I don't like mines like that. AND don't ever do that to me again. Not about food or anything else."

He apologized. But I knew we had no future. *Toys as gifts and control issues were not in my future.*

Once the meal arrived one center piece was well done and the other was medium. I guess the server made her own judgment call. I only ate the piece that came the way that I ordered it.

Over dinner the conversation was little to none. I was still very much irritated. Before I walked out of the restaurant, I called home. My dad answered. "Hey dad. I just want you to know that I'm out with Landon, and I should be home in 30 minutes."

Side Bar: *Ladies and Gentlemen if you find yourself in a situation that you feel uncomfortable in **slow down**. Take a moment and listen to the voice within. If you must: grab a cab, call a friend to pick you up, or do like I did and make that person accountable. Allow them to hear you tell a family member or a friend who you are out with. This story does not turn violent, but I felt the need to say this...*

I thought the silence should have been enough to let him know that I was done. But the next day, he came to my job with another gift.

It was a Mrs. Potato Head.

With such cool confidence as I fussed he said, "Stop fussing and just take it apart."

With his suggestion to take it apart, I thought maybe there was something hiding behind one of the pieces. So I took it apart only to find a blank canvas. I was done!

I found myself tangled in between two different voices from my upbringing. My mom always said "No one has to do anything for you and when someone does you should be appreciative." Grandma Prince says "A bad gift is a gift that a person doesn't want and doesn't need." In that moment I moved forward with Grandma's point of view as I said "What's next Care Bear? My Little Pony? Or maybe She-RA.? What makes you purchase items like this for me? He tried to explain but all I heard was "Blah, Blah, Blah..."

I cut him off mid-sentence and said "Landon, this is not working".

"What do you mean? What did I do wrong?" he asked.

"We are not compatible." Mentally we are on two totally different frequencies." I replied.

Then he said, "I don't understand what the problem is!

"You're childish and controlling," I replied.

He tried to explain even the more. But I had no interest in listening so I said "I hate to cut you off, but I have to get back to my client. I'm sure her dryer will be going off any second now." I tried to return the potato head back to him but he absolutely refused to take it. When I went back to my work station, I gave the toy to Tomorrow. She had a 6 year-old daughter *Melody* who is both my cousin and goddaughter and I suggested she give it to her.

Over the next couple days, he called me a few times but I would not answer. After about a week of calls, I finally answered. "Umm hello?" I said. "Tina, I hope I didn't catch you at a bad time. I wanted to talk. I have had a chance to think about everything that you've said, and you were right. I should not have bought you toys. My goal was to purchase items for you that would allow you to go back to a place in life where your only responsibility was to clean your room, do our homework and to have fun. I'm sorry that the gifts made you upset. May we please sit down and talk? I think we could really be good for one another."

"No. I don't think we would be," I answered.

Tina. Please. You won't regret it." He pleaded.

After hearing *his logic* a part of me felt bad for being so mean. So I apologized for my behavior. However I had no interest in moving forward in a relationship with him.

After he asked me a few more times against my better judgment I agreed to meet for lunch. The reality was, he was buying me toys and although I didn't like the toys I have experienced worst afflictions.

During lunch, he explained himself again.

He began with, "I didn't realize you were judging me. I thought we were having fun and I would like a second chance."

As I listened to him I still couldn't believe he bought me toys. Maybe he dated women that were into those kinds of gifts but I couldn't seem to forget the control he had displayed over dinner. I had heard Dr. Maya Angelou say "*When people show you who they are, believe them*," so when he asked me again for a second chance. I said, "Landon I don't think…"

Immediately, he cut me off before I could finish my sentence and said "You know what? I don't know why I'm even wasting my time with you. I am used to dating beautiful women. Intelligent women, like the ones that I attend Case Western Reserve with. I lowered my standards to date you."

I had a hell of a lot that I wanted to say to him but, wisdom said, "Say nothing."

I raised my index finger to notify the server. When he arrived I said, "We're going to need the check please." The server already had the check in hand. As soon as he laid it on the table, Landon said "I'm not paying for your food either. You can pay for your own food."

Then I laughed. This whole thing felt like I was being *Punked*! I looked around and there was no camera or a crew. I put down thirteen dollars towards the twenty-five dollar bill and then he said "What about the tip?" I gathered my things and walked out of the restaurant. By the time I got halfway to my car he was behind me saying, "You never gave me a second chance. I *deserve* a second chance."

I got in my car and drove off. I could not believe what had just happened. Originally I had turned him down because I wasn't attracted to him. Not one feature. Not his walk. Not his height. Not his style of clothing. Not his texture of hair or his hair cut. Not his smile. NOTHING caught my eye. Landon wasn't just childish, he was controlling, verbally abusive, and possibly bi-polar. I was 26 years old and I had never gone Dutch on a date. Every guy that I had ever gone out with had a policy that my money was no good with them. Even on their birthdays I had to convince them to allow me to pay and I certainly hadn't been insulted to that degree.

As the days passed by, it didn't matter that I hadn't answered his calls and totally avoided him at church. He continued to call my phone. He would leave messages saying, "You never gave me a second chance." He didn't stop harassing me until my father called him. One late night after leaving a church function, as I was driving home, in my rear view mirror I could see that Landon was behind me. My phone rang and it was him so I didn't answer. Finally, after the third call I picked up.

"WHAT?"

"Pull over! We need to talk," he replied.

"No! I'm not pulling over because we have nothing to talk about. Besides you don't live this direction. Why are you following me?" I replied.

"You never gave me a second chance! Pull over now! We need to talk!" he insisted in a very aggressive tone.

"Landon we have nothing to talk about. I'm not pulling over. Good bye!!" and I hung up.

He continued to follow me and to call my phone nonstop.

I was nervous and very uncomfortable. It's been weeks since our last lunch and he has been calling me daily leaving messages on my voicemail saying "you never gave me a second chance. I deserve a second chance" and now it was after midnight and he was following me.

I was on Mayfield Road at the borderline of Lyndhurst and Cleveland Height. In these two suburbs the police will ticket you for doing 40 mph in a 35 mph zone. I was flying down Mayfield doing 60 mph. I hoped to get the attention of a police. He was flying behind me while still calling my phone nonstop. At some point he got caught by a red light. I decided to take side streets hoping to lose him. He would have to be a Cleveland Heights resident to get to my house with the route I took. All the while, he was still blowing up my phone. Each call I sent straight to voicemail. A few minutes later I took a slow turn down my street hoping that he hadn't beat me there. If he had, I was going to head straight to the police station, and from there I would call my parents. Moments after making that right onto our street, I looked in my rearview mirror and I could see a car flying behind me. I knew it was him. I flew up our driveway and ran straight in the house. My dad came running to the back door.

With great concern he asked "What's going on? Why did you pull in the driveway like that? And why did you slam the back door?" I told him what happened and immediately he ran outside.

When he came back in the house he said, "as soon as he saw me he pulled off. Call Him. Now!" So, I did and I put the phone on speaker.

"Landon this is Tina's dad. She told me what just happened." Landon cut him off mid-sentence...

"But, Mr. Lindsey she never gave me second chance!"

"Landon LISTEN! My dad replied, I am only going to tell you this one time. Don't ever call my daughter's phone again. When you see her don't even speak to her, and if you ever follow her again, you will regret it! Do we have a clear understanding?"

That was the end of Landon. But I still changed my phone number.

SO, when Bryant would invite me to comedy shows, concerts, dinner, plays, etc... I had no interest. Thanks for the invite, but no thank you. After Landon,

A BOLD PERSPECTIVE

I was a total skeptic...

After a month or so, of chatting on the phone with Bryant, we began to meet out. Each time we had a blast! Our conversations were great and we shared many laughs. Laughter was something that we both needed and enjoyed. Life granted us a break.

But now, here I was 700 miles away from home. Oddly enough, although I was in a new city by myself...I felt ALIVE! Here was my RESET, and I was ready for what Atlanta had to offer. I took 30 days and just did me! Fortunately, I had saved enough money to pay all my bills for the next 6 months. Therefore, there was no immediate pressure to find a job. I realized my desire to shop was no longer there, either. At this point, I began taking bags of clothes and shoes to the Good Will for needy families. I felt LIBERATED. Atlanta was completely different, but exactly what I needed. Back home, I had my entire family, all my friends and a compact schedule. But my subconscious knew that God wouldn't operate in all my clutter. Back home with life as it was, I could never receive the healing that I was looking for.

Epiphany: *To this very day, I don't care much for the mall or the skating rink. Those places represent false attempts at burying sorrows for me.*

CHAPTER 7

LIFE AS IT WAS

In my down time, which I had plenty of, I spent it reading self-help books and lying quietly. Although, I had a television and a telephone it was rare I utilized them. My focus was on my inner being.

My thoughts consumed me. Who am I now? How am I doing...I mean, really doing? What are my life goals? Do I want to be married? Do I want more children?

The silence became a reprieve, and it was in those moments that I could feel some healing. God had my full attention and at times he would speak directly to me but mostly through my dreams. I found a church to attend fairly quickly, too! Life was smooth sailing for me. The connection with myself and the peace of mind I began to encounter are two reasons why I will forever *love my Peach State*!

Before I knew it I had made it to a full year in Atlanta. My relocation proved to be one of my better life decisions. At one point financially, things got pretty tight. I realized that I needed to put my pride aside and ask for some assistance. I called my dad in tears saying, "I'm on the Titanic and it is going down."

"What are you talking about, girl?" he asked.

"I only have $23 dollars left in my account."

"Okay, Tina you are not on the Titanic and you will not sink! *God will take care of his own.*

Sweetie I got to go. I have some errands to run. I will talk to you later."

A BOLD PERSPECTIVE

I could not believe it! I sat my pride to the side and reached out and was denied. He didn't even ask what my needs were and certainly didn't offer to wire me any money. As I sat in front of Kroger, I cried and said out loud, "I only have twenty three dollars to my name and I'm sinking! Well, at least I paid my rent and my car note." Then I thought about my utilities and they were paid too. So were my credit card bills for the month. Next, I looked down at my gas tank and it was half-*FULL*. I wiped my tears as I realized my only real need for the moment was food.

I quoted the scripture that I have read and heard so many times,

I have never seen the righteous forsaken, nor his seed begging bread. -Psalms 37:25.

I went into the grocery store. I bought a loaf of bread, a pack of deli turkey, a case of water and a box of cereal for the week. I spend $12. I got back in the car and sang JEHOVAH JIREH MY PROVIDER all the way home.

A few days later my dad called me back. He explained his urgency to get off the phone during our last conversation. "It hurt my heart to hear you cry. I wanted to send you money, but if I had done that, it would only be a temporary fix. Instead, wisdom said to sow a seed. The money I would have sent you I sowed it in your name to a charity for needy children and I prayed asking God to bless you."

His seed was honored. Over the next couple of weeks my salon clientele picked up and I had sold another home!

I am systematic by character. A distant zip code only changed my surroundings. My patterns remained the same.

Side Bar: *Wherever I travel to in life, when I arrive to that destination, there I will find me EVERYTHING: mentally, emotionally, spiritually, physically, and financially, that I came with will be there, unless I have changed.*

I found myself stuck in the same cycle, *a fixed schedule*.

Sunday mornings at 7:30 am: climb Stone Mountain.

Sunday 10am: church.

Monday, Tuesday, Wednesday 10am-6pm: real estate office and in the field.

Thursday and Friday: salon all day.

GLORY AND BLUES

Saturday 6am-1pm: salon. Saturday 3-7pm: real estate office and in the field.

I lived in Dunwoody and loved it! It was my type of neighborhood. It had Whole Foods, Trader Joe's, Panera Bread, a fancy Mall, and it was surrounded by great eateries. The community was peaceful, yet vibrant.

I was a realtor at Keller Williams -1st Atlanta. It was located in Sandy Springs, a neighboring suburb to Dunwoody. The office was only 5 minutes away from my apartment. That's a big deal in Atlanta because everything is 15, 20, 30 or 40 minutes away. 1st Atlanta had some real movers and shakers within the office. Kimberly Edmonson quickly became my favorite realtor. She was a pretty white lady with beautiful hues of blonde color in her hair. She was so kind and knowledgeable, and she knew real estate like the back of her hand. One day I went to her private office because I needed some advice. I had a listing appointment that I was very nervous about. Kim offered to go with me to my listing appointment. Together we secured that listing and Kim helped me to take it from listing all the way through to closing! It turns out that the same owner had another home that he needed to sell, which became a win-win for the both of us. Together from just those two homes we sold almost two million dollars in real estate!

Daily, I came to 1st Atlanta in my suit and my pumps. Some days I kept it simple with slacks and a blouse. The days that I wore my Coach pumps I got tons of compliments. They were a total hit in the office! Our team meeting was every Tuesday at 10 am. The meetings were optional, but I had a lot to learn and I was always there. I was originally licensed in Ohio just a few months before relocating to Georgia, but my intentions were to get immediate reciprocity and that's what I did.

One morning while leaving my apartment complex en route to the office I saw a familiar face. I thought my eyes were playing tricks on me. It was Rawls' friend, Will! After I parked my car, we gave each other a big hug that was follow with all the OMGs and questions. You live in Atlanta? In this development? How long have you been here? Why did you leave Cleveland?

That was crazy. I hadn't seen him in about 5 years, but whenever I did, he was always so kind to me. He used to work at my favorite furniture store, Seaman's. He even allowed me to use his discount to purchase both my bedroom and living room sets. Before we parted ways I had to ask him "how's Rawls?"

"He's great!" he replied.

"Well tell him I said hello! I have to get to work. It was great seeing you!"

I understand that time and chance happens to us all. But wow! Atlanta is HUGE! With apartment complexes everywhere, yet Will and I end up living in the same complex, in the same timing, just three buildings apart.

Now the salon, that was all together a different experience. I started out looking for an upscale salon, but what I got was a fun and lively salon in the hood. Here's the story. My pastor back at home suggested that I visit his friend's church. He believed that Pastor O'Sneed would be a great shepherd for me, so straight away I visited his church. I had heard him preach a time or two, but back home at a recent women's conference one of his minister's Bernice Davis, preached at our church. She was all of amazing and I wanted to be where I could hear her preach again and again. (Not only did she preach candidly, she was kind hearted too. I was her transport from the airport to the service and then to her hotel. On that day she deposited spiritual jewels into my life.)

As soon as he saw me he said, "Hey! Don't I know you?"

"Yes." I replied.

Back home, because I was the first lady's armor-bearer, at church I was always found sitting on the front row, to the immediate right or left of the pastor's wife. When special guest were in town for a conference a catered dinner was at their home and I would assist. Pastor O'Sneed had been a guest preacher several times. So it was no surprise he had recognized me. I explained to him that I had just recently moved to the city.

"Do you need anything?" he asked.

"Yes," I replied. "A referral! I'm looking for a salon to work in." I gave him my whole spiel. "I want to work in an *upscale salon with high-end clientele*, maybe in Sandy Springs or one of the neighboring suburbs."

In mid-sentence he said, "I got something for you! Call up here to the church tomorrow afternoon. I'll have to contact the owner first..."

I did as instructed. He let me know he had arranged an interview for the following morning. He gave me the address and said, "I'll meet you there!" I was too excited, until I pulled up to the building and realized it was in the center of the hood. If I weren't meeting the pastor there I would have kept going. I parked my car and fussed to myself, "what part of upscale salon in the suburbs did he not understand?"

  Finally I went inside of the salon. The owner was short in height but lofty in personality. He was a Jamaican man by the name of Rich. He was very excited about his business and he should have been because it was actually a nice salon. He had 12 stylists, 4 barbers (including himself) and a nail tech. The Pastor said he had another salon that was located a mile down the road and it was similar in size. This salon didn't match what I was looking for, but Rich made me an offer I couldn't refuse. Free booth rent for 1 month! That was unheard of. It wasn't normal practice for him to offer such a deal. Rich didn't offer commission and I only had one client, Kelli who had just moved from Cleveland too.

Right away I got busy passing out flyers. I would pass them out almost every place that I went. All the ladies at Pastor O's church got one. Before I knew it 4 members from the church became my regular clients: Tiffanie, Stephanie, Latonia, and Alexis. I didn't remain at that church but I was glad that I followed the instruction of my previous Pastor.

The salon was high energy. People interacted with each other, laughed and cracked jokes all day. My station was the very last station in the back, which was a catch 22. Walk-ins came in everyday but none made it all the way to the back, unless all of the other stylists were too busy to take them, or Rich grabbed them and sent them my way. That was the down side. The up side was, in the back we had a lot of fun because we had our own little section. In the beginning most days were awkward because everyone was busy but me. I could remember my Abracadabra Salon days being like that. Back home we were busy from the time we walked in the door until the time we left. If and when you ate lunch, it was inhaled. I understood that it is a process to build a clientele. If I bid my time, built my brand with persistence and consistency, within a few months I could have a steady flow once again.

Just like that it happened. My business had begun to grow.

One day, which wasn't uncommon for me to have a still moment, I sat in my chair waiting for my client to arrive. The barber who worked across from me was sitting too which was weird because he was always busy. RA's grooming chair stayed loaded, but in that moment he too was in wait of his next client.

"So Tina, where you from?" RA asked.

"*Cleveland,*" I replied.

"Where you from?"

"*Philly*," he replied.

"What brought you here?" he asked me.

"I just needed something different. I couldn't do the snow and brutal cold anymore, and I wanted to be in a city that was vibrant. Every time I came here to visit I just liked it. Besides, I needed a new start!"

"What do you mean a new start?" he asked.

Not sure what made me tell him, but I did. "I lost my son some years back. Everything at home reminded me of him and everyone knew what happened to me. I just needed to get away."

He sat there speechless. Until that very moment we had only had group conversations which were mostly joke related.

A month or so later we had another downtime moment. This time there was no need for the previous where you from... we had already had that exchange. He asked me "have you ever heard the song "Let it Burn...you know the Usher song?"

I gave the dumbest response, "yeah back home they used to play that song all day on the radio. It was played at least three times a day."

To myself all I could think was, "Really, Tina? All day? Three times? Please think before you speak. Ugh!"

"Well, I'm thinking about letting it burn," he said.

Because I knew the lyrics and I had seen his wife in the salon a few times, I knew what his statement meant, so I went into fix-it mode.

"Well, maybe together, y'all can read a book on marriage. Then discuss the chapters together."

He closed his eyes, mildly shook his head and then said "Nah, that won't work."

I followed with "Okay so maybe counseling will work."

He replied, "Nah. That won't work either. We have passed all fixing points."

That explained why over the last few weeks he hadn't seemed himself. At least not the person I had originally met. He used to come to work early in the morning cracking jokes. Lately it had taken him a while to warm up. Even once he warmed up he still wasn't the same.

After a year of working at Rich's Salon I had built a decent clientele, but I was ready to get back to my original vision of working in an upscale salon. Unlike before where my sights were only set on the northern section of the city, I had a new desire to work in the city's center, Midtown. One day while at work I shared my plans with my immediate neighbors RA and Summer. To my surprise Summer was on her way out the door to fill a management position at a salon in a nearby mall, and RA had plans to open a salon in midtown. After a few detailed conversations RA asked me to join his business venture. He offered me a management position with 10% ownership. Of course I accepted the offer. I didn't have to bring any capital, just management responsibilities and salon expertise. Straight away I began researching salon equipment, startup costs, policy procedure manuals, etc. At work I would deliver my findings to him.

Life was looking good! I had taken a chance by relocating miles away from home. By the end of the first year my salon clientele had a steady flow. I had sold 5 homes, even though two of my closings almost fell through. My co-worker Mahogany Rhodes helped me to hold those deals together with her infamous business model MO Knows Real Estate.

Oh yeah, I had a little friend too! Daily we met at The Breakfast Cafe'. My life was so systematic that after a few weeks the chef had me memorized. Within minutes of scoring our table our server would deliver my freshly squeezed O.J with my waffle and omelet with mushrooms, onions, peppers, turkey and cheddar cheese. After breakfast, off to work he went and so did I.

STONE MOUNTAIN

One Monday morning I woke up very unsettled. I had missed my mountain workout. Every Sunday morning before church Erica (Will's wife) and I would climb to the top of Stone Mountain. After our workout we would rush home and shower up for church. This particular Sunday she wasn't available. It was Monday and I felt like the rest of my week would be doomed if I didn't stick to my routine, so I decided to call her.

A BOLD PERSPECTIVE

"Hey Erica! You want to go to the mountain today?"

"I wish I could but I have to work late tonight." she replied.

Next I called Mary aka Mai. She and I used to work together at Abracadabra Salon and she also lived in Atlanta. My first Stone Mountain experience was with her. But she was unavailable too.

I thought about asking my breakfast date, but I knew that would be a waste of breath. Everywhere we went he valeted. He said it was because he didn't want anyone to put a dent in his Range or his Benz, which might ring some truth, but I think it was because he was lazy too. I thought briefly about going alone but that thought didn't settle well. As I was sitting there pondering about what I should do next, I had a light bulb moment! RA was always talking about working out and how he goes running, so I called him.

"Hey RA! How are you doing today?"

"I'm alright," he said.

"I have an idea! I think you should get out and get some fresh air today."

"What do you mean?" he asked.

"I'm walking Stone Mountain about 11ish. You should come," I replied.

"Umm NO," he said.

"I have a lot to do this morning. I have to do some banking, paying bills and I have a meeting," he explained.

"Alright then. I just thought you could use the fresh air." Dang, I couldn't get anybody to go with me.

It was now five o'clock and I decided that I was going even if it meant going alone. Before heading out I decided to give it one more shot. I made one last phone call.

"Hey RA! This is Tina again."

"What's up Tina?" he asked.

I replied "This morning you said no to going to the mountain because you had banking and other business stuff to do. Now, all those places are closed. I'll be honest. I don't want to go by myself, but I do think you could use some fresh air too."

I waited in silence.

After breathing hard he said, "Alright I'll go."

I replied, "*Kool Beanz*!!! Let's meet at 6:30."

He showed up in a funk! Like I had forced him to do something against his will. *Maybe I kind of did*, but I was glad that I didn't have to walk this mountain alone. This was his first time walking Stone Mountain. I had completed this climb every Sunday morning for the past two months, but for whatever the reason on this particular day I was so winded. I had to sit down and sip my water a couple of times. Each time he stared at me as if he wanted to say REALLY?

Finally on my third sit down he said it. "You harassed me about coming to this mountain and now I have to keep waiting on you!"

"I'm sorry. This doesn't normally happen," I replied. I gathered myself and proceeded on. Once we made it to the top of the mountain the breeze and the view were breath taking. The energy of nature was totally different in the evening than in the morning. We took a seat on a stone that faced the city while we caught our breath. We talked about Atlanta, the future salon endeavor, our childhood[s], life goals and failures, value systems, the guy that I was dating, the loss of my son, and his dreams and concerns for his children. He even told me why he was getting a divorce.

I can't remember who said it, but one of us said it was time to go. We turned around to leave and it was pitch black. Looking out towards the city was all lights. Behind us, which was the direction to exit the mountain, it was total darkness. We could barely see two feet ahead of us. We were so engaged in our conversation, we didn't realize that the sun and all the other climbers had left. I was terrified. RA quickly took charge.

"Do you know which direction we need to go?" he asked.

I replied "Yes to the right. I can direct us, but please don't let me fall. I trip during the day on some of these stones and right now I can barely see them."

He said okay and extended his hand. My hesitancy must have spoken volumes because next he said, "Tina, I'm not trying to make a move on you. I was just trying to do what I think is best to assist you."

"Thanks, but no thanks. I'll just hold onto your arm." I replied.

What I didn't know was under all those 3X baggy t-shirts was actually a firm bicep. I grabbed his arm and immediately let go.

He laughed and said, "Ah! She didn't know that was there!" and we both laughed.

We slowly walked forward. I tripped a few times but I never fell because each time he caught me. As we approached some of the larger stones he would say "wait, let me step down first." He would then take my hand and assist me. I didn't resist, as safety became top of the agenda. The journey down felt like forever. When we finally saw the light ahead we turned to each other. I was going to say "we made it!"

We were stuck in a daze into each other's eyes. In silence we both turned forward adding a little distance in between us and continued the odyssey.

Once we reached our cars RA asked, "*Would you like to get some ice cream or coffee?*" "Yes I would!" I answered. I had a thing for cookies and cream ice cream.

As I ate my ice cream and he sipped on his coffee, we sat on the hood of my car and conversed for another hour. Eventually we went our separate ways. The evening was magical. It was as if we were hit by Cupid's bow. We went up the mountain one way and came down another way, but we didn't discuss it. There were red flags everywhere.

A. RA had become my friend and there was no need in messing up a good friendship.

B. He and his wife were separated, but the divorce was not finalized.

C. I won't be nobodies rebound. Fresh out of a marriage… that's all that I would be. So friends we would remain.

Most of the time RA and I would have discreet conversations at work about the future salon plans. I can remember a time or two where we met at a bookstore. Once we even met at a salon equipment store. In all of our chatting, we never discussed the mountain. It was business and life conversations as usual.

A few weekends later, RA asked me if I could help him with his daughter's hair. It was his weekend to have the kids and according to him, "her hair was in need of a little assistance." RA was in the industry, but mainly as a barber. His hair game was limited to male grooming. After finishing his daughter's hair he tried to compensate me but I refused his pay. So he invited me to go skating

GLORY AND BLUES

with him and the kids and I accepted. I had a lot fun! I hadn't been skating in years. His children Tashon, Jasrah, and Jamal were all very sweet too.

Several more months had gone by and I was more than ready to leave the south side of town. RA's salon was still an unfinished project and his business partner was unsure about a three-way partnership so, I split. I found a beautiful salon to work in and it was located in midtown. From the outside looking in Salon Lotus was all of that. But, the business had two partners. One partner was a great stylist who worked in the salon with us. She was sweet and very talented. In many ways she reminded me of my favorite stylist Tammy Cartwright from home. Tammy and I worked together at Abracadabra for 7 years. Hands down everything from skill sets, to personality to fashion Tammy had it! In all my years of styling, I have yet to work with a more well rounded stylist. Oh yeah, did I mention that she was as cute as a button? She looks like the black light-skinned version of Punky Buster. Tammy is a pure beauty with a face full of freckles!

Back to the midtown salon… The other partner had invested the majority of the capital and she ran the business in arrogance. Basic things like lighting she didn't seem to understand or care about. Without the proper lighing, a stylist would be unable to see their client's hair color. Even though it was a simple fix of swapping a 40watt light for a 75watt light. There were a few other things that I was dissatisfied with but I dismissed them. What I couldn't dismiss was the fact that every Saturday the receptionist would be late. Sometime 10 minutes. Sometimes 20 minutes. She was the key holder and we could not enter the building until she arrived. The ownership acted as if it was no big deal. After a couple months of that foolishness I left.

RA and his business partner had finally opened Dream Salon so, I joined the team. Dream was alluring with hardwood flooring, white decor and red accents. My clients loved it and so did I!

As some point, RA asked me to meet him at Barnes and Noble on Peachtree Rd. That day we had *the* conversation. He was available… and so was I, but there was still more things to discuss. We had become great friends and our dating would result in ALL or NOTHING. If we gave it a shot and it didn't work we could never go back, so we had a serious decision to make and that day we decided…*All!*

On our first date we grabbed a bite to eat at a casual restaurant. We talked for hours. While out to dinner his mom called. Within moments of their conversation he said "my mom would like to speak with you." She started the exchange with "I am so happy to speak with you! I have heard great things about you and I can't wait to meet you!" I returned pleasantries and then handed RA back his cell phone. To myself I thought, "Wow. He told his mom about me!"

In the early stages of our relationship we spent hours discussing our childhood dreams, adult goals, morals, world affairs, and life. Our conversations were rarely about us as a couple. We spent time listening to one another and building each other up as individuals. Through friendship we created a rock solid bond. We were confidantes and stood in the gap for each other. Not to mention we had so much in common! We shared core values and perspectives. He was easy going...like the yen to my yang.

But for me I was behind the eight ball. You see girls, we got game too! I had been sharing my game with him when I was going to him for advice for my little breakfast date. Looking back retrospectively, I think RA advised me out of my relationship. I'm glad that he did, but in the interim he was learning my game and my strategies.

After a year and some change of dating, we decided to take a vacation. The morning of the flight RA called me and asked me, "Are you watching the news?"

"No I'm not" I replied.

He said. "Well, cars are floating down the streets of Miami. You should turn the news on." I did and cars were floating just like he said.

I called the airline and the flight wasn't cancelled, so I called him back and said, "We're going..." As we sat in the airport the television screens showed the same pictures of cars floating down the street. "Tina! I don't think we should we go. This is ridiculous!" he said.

"We'll be fine RA!" I replied. I was determined to go. I was in need of a vacation.

He shook his head almost the entire flight, but no way was he going to allow me to go alone and I was going with or without him. One hour and twenty-five minutes later, we arrived in Miami. We didn't see any floating cars, just a light drizzle. We caught a cab to our Ocean Drive hotel and within minutes the strip was infused with the radiance of sunshine.

GLORY AND BLUES

The first night we went to Tropical Cafe, a swanky lounge on the South Beach strip. Downstairs we had dinner and we watched the live band and dancers perform on the bar top. At some point we made our way upstairs to the dance floor. The DJ was jamming and so were we! We danced the night away or at least tried to, as I was giving RA and the dance floor everything that I had. I noticed the girl next to me was almost taken down by a huge pillow. She and I were both very confused as we stopped dancing and stared at the pillow that was now lying on the floor beside us. I saw a second pillow fly across the room and it hit another person. By that point I was totally scanning the room and there they were. Three huge muscle bound Latino men. They were throwing pillows from off the couch and with each contact they laughed. RA grabbed my hand and said, "Let's go. If they hit me or you with one of those pillows my pride won't let me just walk away....

There's three of them and one of me..." So we left. The muscle-bound overstuffed kids wrecked our jam zone.

The second day after being at the beach for many hours we decided to shower up and get dressed. As we walked the ocean's shore the sky opened up and it began to rain. We ran into the closest booth for shelter. The life guard looked onto an empty beach. Everyone had run off and he did the same as he said, "It's all yours!"

Out in the ocean was a ship that had been in that same spot since we arrived. I said, "Look RA that's the same ship from yesterday. I wonder why it's just sitting in the center of the ocean. Then he said "It looks like that ship has planted its anchor. It's about time I plant mines. I want you to be my wife."

Out of his pocket he pulled out a small box. "Will you be my wife?" he asked.

"YES! I will!" I gladly replied.

Suddenly, a lady and her daughter ran into our booth. I couldn't resist. I needed my "Instagram moment". "Would you please take a picture of us?" I asked.

She did. After she handed me back my phone she and her daughter ran off into the rain. Within seconds the sun came back out. Hand in hand we walked off into the sunlight. "So, RA did you plan the rain too?" I asked, and he responded with a smile.

CHAPTER

8

NOTEBOOK

Chicken and scalloped potatoes were baking in the oven as I prepped my salad. A little reggae music was playing in the back ground and RA was in a zone. Like usual, RA had come to my house for dinner. I could hear him on the phone. "Listen Man, in this world you have to *empower yourself.* No one is going to just give you power. *Power is only taken.*" He must have been on the phone with President Obama, shortly after Health Care Reform was finalized.

While I was enjoying the atmosphere my cell phone rang and I answered. "Hello?"

"May I speak to Tina?" the voice said.

Right away I knew who it was.

"This is Tina." I slowly replied.

"Hey this is Rawls. I hope you don't mind me calling you. I got your number from Will. I've been wanting to call you for quite a while, but first I wanted to wait until my divorce was final and now it is. You have always stayed with me. I guess it's safe to say it wasn't over for me."

Here I stood in a real life NOTEBOOK moment, just like in one of my favorite movies. I was now engaged and the man whom I never stopped loving had just resurfaced.

As he continued on, I disappeared into my grey matter. There was no bad decision to be made here. They would both love me. Both roads would lead to happiness.

Rawls had jumped in the fiery furnace with me. In one year without thought he was fired from four jobs. All in the name of, "*I gotta see about my girl.*" To him I mattered and everyday he showed it. He brought calm to the toughest year of my life. His chivalry was to be studied. In our year of dating, I never opened one car door.

RA had stretched me. Because of him I really believed that my only limitations were in my mind. My dad says, ["Tina? Now she has a fixed heart and a made up mind. Once she decides on something that is it. Your only shot is to get to her before she makes a decision."] That is so true about me but RA was the exception though. He had changed my mind many times. Together we had some of the most mentally stimulating conversations and our friendship was incredible. I loved RA and I knew he loved me too.

But I also loved Rawls. Prior to this phone call I had no doubts about me and RA. Instantly, I began to wonder if I was making the right decision. If life took a second emotional turn would RA comfort me like Rawls had?

I knew that this would probably be the most important natural life decision that I would make. Whichever road I took would alter my course forever.

As Rawls continued to speak, I looked up at RA and he smiled at me. He had a sparkle in his eyes that wasn't there before. We had been together for almost two years, but I had known him for four years now. In his "*right now*" reality he was on fire for life. With RA and I, we weren't just a couple. We were friends. *And friends don't hurt friends.* On top of that, I couldn't imagine my future without RA as my life partner, coach and friend. Finally I spoke.

"I'm getting married in 60 days."

I didn't sleep at all that night or the next, or even the next night after that.

CHAPTER 9

SECOND CHANCE

On a chilly fall night, under the moonlit sky in a gazebo dressed in chiffon and all white lights, we said *I Do*!

My Auntie Rosemary and my father united us in matrimony. I married a tall, handsome, gentleman by the name of Rashon D. Fuller. He is my spoken word; my rhythmic poetry; my inspiration for *self-articulation*; he is my wow and my encore!

Rashon and I were told by many couples that the first year of marriage would be the toughest year. Yet, we breezed right through it! Our relationship was full of laughter, understanding, dancing, many smiles and much communication. However, the second year was a different story.

At 30, one year prior to marriage, I decided I didn't want more children. Well, I didn't really decide, I allowed FEAR to decide. I grappled with the thought of losing another child or not loving a future child like I loved Kevin. I believed I would always be on the edge, extremely emotional and overprotective.

One day, I was enraged. It was a normal practice for me to call my father when I was battling decisions because I knew he would listen, then pray for me and offer sound advice. So, I called him. I told him I didn't want any more children! There was a silent pause, and then he lovingly said "That's fine but don't make that decision from this position. Tina, you are only 32 years old. I want you to go down the road…travel to age 60. If at that age you don't want any children or grandchildren visiting you, especially on the holidays, then proceed without having children. But, if you may want that, then now is the time!"

My dad and his words always have a way of making me put things in proper perspective. That evening, I came home with 2 ovulation predictors! The first test showed positive for a LH surge! I was ready to try but something strange happened. We didn't use any protection that cycle or the next and we didn't conceive. In my family if you think about sex (without protection), then BOOM... you're pregnant!

After a few months of not conceiving, I began to do research about natural fertility remedies. The most successful remedy was DIET. I learned my diet should consist of lots of raw, fresh vegetables and fruits, nuts, seeds, natural fats, multi-vitamins, lots of water and moderation of animal products. In conjunction avoiding anti-nutrients: high fructose corn syrup (HFCS), processed foods, etc. RA and I quickly jumped into this new lifestyle.

A year passed and we still had not conceived. After that year of TTC (trying to conceive) that's when we discovered just how emotionally unstable I was. I became distraught and impulsive. I implored defense mechanisms and put up walls to protect myself emotionally. Many days, my husband was confused, irritated, and provoked. In spite of all of this, Rashon loved me through it. His love and commitment to me meant more to him than my impulsive dysfunction.

In our 2nd year of TTC we began fertility testing. My GYN did all the basics for fertility testing. Rashon was immediately excluded as his results scored high. After being unable to identify a problem we were referred to a specialist. However, through an untrasound my doctor did discover that I had 3 fibroids. One the size of a plum and two the size of a pea. I chose not to go to the specialist straight away. I decided to research natural remedies for fibroids. The diets were very similar to the suggested fertility diets. For the next six months we continued with my holistic journey, which I call *Endo-Boost*.

After six more months, I looked and felt amazing. My body had taken on a new slender shape. I was also experiencing high levels of energy and alertness, but still no conception. So I went to the specialist, an endocrinologist. To my surprise my largest fibroid that was the size of a plum had shrank down to the size of a cherry! My progesterone levels had increased from 7.5 to 12! After viewing my records and not being able to identify a problem she began more advanced testing.

Over the course of a year I took three (HSG's) Hysterosalpingograms a x-ray test that evaluates the inside of the uterus and the fallopian tubes. With the first two tests they couldn't tell if the tubes were open or closed.

OCTOBER 24th 2012

This day marked one of the saddest days of my life. The comprehension of my son's death didn't happen in one day. My body's natural intelligence cultivated a lapse of solidity. Psychologically, I was numb, but this report came with no filter. Immediately I was devastated. Here I was **R-E-A-D-Y** *for my second chance* and both of my fallopian tubes were blocked.

Tremendous despair flooded my total being. My doctor's suggestion was to get laparoscopy to confirm the blockage, and after that we could better assess the best method for in vitro fertilization (IVF). But she made it very clear that in order to avoid the risk of a tubal pregnancy, my fallopian tubes would have to be removed.

While walking stone-faced through the parking garage of the doctor's office, Rashon grabbed my hand and said "STOP. *Just stop*." He grabbed me in his arms and held me and I wept. He said "I know what the results were. But I have faith that God will bless us with children. We are going to stand on The Rock (Our Creator)!"

His words were comforting, but I was hurt beyond measure. I cried nonstop for hours.

Later that evening I informed Rashon and my doctor that I would take a nine month break to work on me. My plan moving forward was to continue with the "*endo-boost*" plus incorporate a consistent regiment of prayer, yoga, meditation, acupuncture, and to pay off the remaining balance of the five thousand dollars in medical expenses that we had accumulated during fertility testing.

Side Bar: *Assisted Reproductive Technology (ART) is a beautiful and fascinating science. Countless families have accomplished their dreams of parenthood through this science. However, we didn't feel that IVF was the strategy for us. (At least not just yet) The fact that the natural course of procreation was not taking place, allowed us to know that the body lacked harmony and balance. We didn't want to shortcut our imbalance. Our target was to correct it, naturally. When the body is out of balance it causes weakness and that weakness is absorbed within the total anatomy. Our goal was to strengthen our core.*

I decided that no one would be removing my tubes! For me the removal of my tubes was like removing God out of the equation, and I had no interest in being at the total mercy of science.

Believe it or not, I tackled my plan with vigilance, but emotionally I was out of control. Being married to me during that time, had to be equivalent to being with a person with *emotional dementia*. I was up and down, in and out. Seriously, I was a wreck and we both knew it. It seemed like all the emotions surrounding Kevin's death had resurfaced. I reached a place where I couldn't determine if I was hysterical due to his death, fertility challenges or both. *And that wasn't all.* I'm sweet, silly, and kind by nature. However, LOVE was no longer easy for me. Saying the "L" word became extremely difficult. I would cringe when people would say it to me because that meant I was obligated to say it back. Yes, it affected our marriage, too. I couldn't explain what was happening and Rashon constantly wanted to discuss what was going on. "Tina there is an elephant in the room and it's too big to ignore." Each attempt at discussing this felt like another lecture.

I loved my husband, and I trusted him. However, I wanted to stay where I wasn't obligated to love deeply and it was a major cause of friction. Rashon wanted us to love one another without limits, but I didn't have it in me. I was full of limitations…most of them I didn't even know existed until they showed up. In a normal functioning relationship, love grows and the couple advances to the next level. Rashon and I would advance. The moment that I realized we had gone a little higher I was instantly uncomfortable and I would retreat. Emotionally I would rebuild my walls. My thoughts were what if he ends up in a car accident or something and dies? I haven't recovered from the first heartbreak. Truth is, *I was married but afraid to love.*

It had been nine months and two weeks since my last HSG. I had reached an all-time low. I could no longer stand in the gap for me. Emotionally and mentally I had given life everything that I had. Not just with this whole fertility thing, but even dating back to Kevin's death. For many years I had carried a longing hurt and it was still so intense. Within its core was tremendous anger. It was just too much and I had reached my *Breaking Point*.

THE BREAKING POINT

I stood in the mirror trying to see into the heart of my soul. My mind wasn't ready to quit, but my eyes revealed that all my strength was gone. I had no fight left. I only had my feet that I stood on, my hands which were raised in total surrender, and my voice that cried out "**GOD, You forgot about me.**"

I began to sing an old *hymn*

PASS ME NOT O GENTLE SAVIOUR,

Hear my humble cry;

While on others Thou art calling,

Do not pass me by.

What seems like only moments later, my Aunt Lauretta called, "Tina I know you don't know this lady, but I do! Her name is Vera. She just called me and said, The Lord has a word for you. She wants you to call her."

So, of course, I asked "How do you know the word is for me?" My aunt replied, "Her description matches you. Call me when you get off the phone with her. I want to know what she said."

I was hesitant, for many reasons. First, I was not in the mood, second, I didn't know her, and finally, I was supposed to call a lady in a nursing home on her cell phone, really?

I don't know why I even answered the phone. Certainly today was so not a good day for this, but out of respect and obedience for my aunt I called her.

"Hello, may I speak with Ms. Vera?" I said.

"Speaking", she replied.

"This is Tina I said, Lauretta's niece." She didn't waste a minute. She went straight to it. "Baby, God said *He has not forgotten about you*. God said that you have been unhappy for quite a while. God said that you are about to experience a level of love that you have never experienced before. God said that he is going to restore you, **-*but first you must share your story.*** You must tell your testimony."

TESTIMONY??? This is not a testimony. This is a mess, I thought to myself.

I began to weep because God HEARD ME, and because I didn't want to publicly share *things* that had caused me tremendous grief.

Ms. Vera asked, "Baby, are you crying?" I got just enough voice to say "Yes." She then replied, "Let me pray." The more she prayed, the harder I cried. After a few minutes I was sobbing like a lost child. She said "Hold on baby let me put my prayer partner on the phone, she wants to pray too." At some point while they were both praying on the speaker phone, pride and embarrassment kicked in and I said "Thank you, thank you so much but I have to go now."

I hung up the phone but I couldn't rejoice. I was clouded by two words: *share* and *testimony*. I knew that I had experienced a divine encounter because I had just said "God, you forgot about me." Even the words that followed defined my life completely, but the thought of humiliation by way of self-exposure was too much to ask.

After I calmed myself, I call Auntie Lauretta back. As I conveyed all that was said to me, I was enraged by the time I got to that "t" word. "This is a mess! There is no testimony to be told here!" Again I began to cry. Right away she replied "Tina, I remember years ago as you and I sat solo on a bench in the church foyer, with a radiant glow you said, "Auntie! I had lost my mind and God gave it back to me!" "That is a testimony!" she replied and continued, "Most people don't get their minds back after they lose it. She then asked, what has you so upset today?" I began telling her about my fertility challenges.

"Oh honey, I had no idea. I just thought you and RA decided not to have kids. I'm so sick of this Devil. Let's pray." she said and she did...

After we hung up the phone, I called my father. He answered and I began telling him about my conversation with Ms. Vera. In the spirit of confusion I proceeded, "I don't see a testimony. I'm living in a nightmare. What is there to share? How can this story help anyone?"

Calmly he said "Well-Tina I recently shared the story of how my grandson was hit and killed by a car. I told them the girl who hit him was contemplating suicide. I continued telling them how you called that girl over to our house and held her in your arms. You restored hope back into that young lady's life. Today, she is alive because of you. "Sweetie, you DO have a testimony and it restored hope to a group of hopeless people!

He continued, I know how much you loved Kevin and you were an amazing mother to him. After he died I was afraid. I didn't know if emotionally you could sustain such a devastating blow. I feared what would become of you. With a close eye I watched and prayed for you. You have made me so very proud. With a pen and paper I could not have written a better story about a mother who lost her son."

Needless to say, I cried even more. After those three phone calls I was drained spiritually, mentally, physically and emotionally. My sentiments hadn't budged concerning the testimony. I had no interest in sharing stories that I worked so hard to conceal. Sixteen years later and I could barely think about Kevin without becoming emotionally overwhelmed, let alone talk about him. I lived my life trying not to think about him or what had happened. I didn't then and still don't allow my family to talk about him in my presence. My fertility challenges were personal and extremely humiliating, so much so, that the majority of my family didn't even know about my challenges. So, the idea of sharing these stories troubled me.

CHAPTER 10

UNTITLED

If my audience were from Cleveland I would say "He was the Coventry type." If my audience were from Atlanta, I would say "You know... the Little Five Points type." White guy, super painted pale skin with piercing and tattoos everywhere. Black hair, black clothes, black shoes, he even carried a black backpack. This guy was totally all black and all white. I can't remember his name but my first year of college I had a class with him. At this stage I can't remember which class, but that isn't important. He was always very quiet, yet very intense. Whenever I saw him in the cafeteria he was alone. A few times, I took a seat at his the table where he sat solo (I was quite social back then). He always looked at me and smiled, and in return I'd say, "Hey! How are ya?" While chatting he never laughed much but at least I made him smile. One Wednesday evening while I was at home praying, God spoke to me in an audible voice and gave me a word to share with him.

The next day when I saw him, as always he was alone. As I contemplated telling him I was over taken by fear. I thought to myself, he is going to think I'm weird. I chickened out and proceeded to walk in the opposite direction. "God I'm sorry. I just couldn't do it. I'll tell him tomorrow. I promise." As I walked through the hall to my next class I felt bad. When I got home I felt worst. I was given an assignment and I failed. I had failed God.

As I was getting dressed for school the next morning, he was on my mind. With a solid plan, I decided, if he thinks that I'm weird so be it. The moment I laid eyes on him, I would tell him what the Lord said. That day, he didn't come to class and he wasn't in the cafeteria either. As I looked for him my guilt intensified. I couldn't find him and I never saw him again. That day I made God a promise. "If you ever tell me to tell anyone, anything else, I will!" Well... God never asked me to deliver another word until Ms. Vera...

For the next three days, I complained to myself; both out loud and in my head. Eventually I expressed my frustration to Rashon. "God is a Bully! Do you think Jonah wanted to be in the belly of that whale? Don't answer, it's rhetorical. Of course he didn't. *But* all because he didn't tell the people of Nineveh what God said, he was swallowed by a whale!"

On the sixth day, as I sat at a red light, I looked up towards the sky and said "GOD this story is humiliating! To share it exposes me and I am emotionally introverted. WHY would you ask me to share this story?" I proceeded, "The story should go like this, after the death of my two year old son and in the face of fertility challenges, I used God's remedies to heal my body and guess what, we're expecting! But NO God, *this story is incomplete*!"

Then he finally spoke in an audible voice, "**THAT'S THE BEAUTY OF IT.**"

His tone was as *peaceful* and *calming* as it was *that day* in the basement in the *tarrying room*.

After the light turned green I proceeded home. Upon arriving, I immediately placed myself in front of the mirror, the same one that I saw defeat in just six days ago. This time I saw me differently. Beyond the tears that flowed like a river, there was hope, acceptance and finally *surrender*. Somewhere in between the words from Ms. Vera and God speaking to me at the stop light, I had embodied a *spiritual evolution*; fear had scattered and faith had taken over. For whatever reason, it was my social *responsibility* to share my story and the time had come.

Life had shown me that it's impossible for fear and faith to share one space, as one will take over the other. My heart and mind settled on faith.

Though he slay me, **YET WILL I TRUST HIM**. -Job 13:15.

WALKING OUT THE PROCESS

I realized that in order to share my story, I would have to go back to my earliest memories; so that's what I did. I started at about 5 years old playing with my sister Kisha and my cousin Tomorrow. I was the most sensitive kid ever and they knew it. The two of them constantly terrorized me. They would pick up anything (a rock, a piece of lint, a broken toy, dirt, a dead bug, etc…) and say, "This is what your kids are going to look like!" They would laugh and I would cry, kick and scream.

From there, I journeyed on to my childhood fears. I was terrified of those big characters at the amusement parks: Mickey Mouse, Donald Duck, Care Bears, all of them. My belief was that anything that big should not be walking and talking.

I remembered being eight years old with a real passion for Christ.

I thought about all the nights that I spent over my Auntie Jewel's house. Some summers, I spent practically the entire vacation over my aunts' home. Her home was like Disney World. Not just for me and all my cousins but for the neighborhood kids too. In her home, there were not just her children, but their friends and family members also. The guys would be out back playing basketball with her son, Omega. The girls were in the house getting all dolled up to go to the mall. Auntie Jewel would always pull me and her daughter, Chiron to the side and ask "you girls have enough money?" We always said "No!" She would go in her tiny black coach purse and pull out several twenties. In the nineties as a teenager, having $40 to go shopping was a big deal! Me and my cousins Chiron, Omega, Jamal, and Jae, would stay up playing cards all night.

I thought about school and *all* of my friendships throughout the years.

My mental odyssey landed me at 15 years old and in a relationship with Mylon. I thought about all the walks to class and through the park. We spent senseless hours on the phone talking about everything and nothing at all. I stopped there and decided that I would pick back up the next day. I had spent hours reliving the first half of my life and emotionally I was wiped-out.

The next morning I picked up right where I left off. Quickly, I saw myself 16 years old and pregnant. The day before, as I reminisced, it was with smiles and laughter. Today it was serious; no smiles and no laughter. The turning point in my life started with pregnancy. I didn't shy away either; I embodied all the emotions. I felt like I was 16 years old and pregnant again. I relived the shame and anger.

Then the labor hit. After Kevin was born I stared into his eyes again. Time stood still and I found a piece of me. I stayed in that moment until the daze faded away.

It was time to continue on.

I traveled back to high school after my maternity leave. Shortly after, I graduated from high school. This time, I was proud of me! It wasn't easy balancing being a teenager, a mom with so much responsibility, business clientele and having to study, but I did it!!! Like dad had said… and I finished school on time! I walked the stage as a Cleveland Heights High School Graduate with the Class of 1996!

I thought about Kevin's first haircut with his 1st barber Tommy. I listened to him scream like someone was killing him.

My thoughts journeyed back to my freshman year at Cuyahoga Community College aka TRI-C. I realized that I *owe* Dion some gas money for him picking me up for school every day. He never asked for a dime or anything in return. I thought about my classmate Olivia Watson who I attended both Heights High and TRI-C with. On several occasions, she drove me home when Dion had to leave early.

I remembered how my favorite courses were communication classes. I always looked forward to and excelled in those classes.

Then, I saw myself in the cafeteria checking on Dion as he stood by the elevator in a daze. This time instead of Dion's eyes being fixated on the man in the all black suit and the white clergy, *my eyes were fixated.*

As the minister spoke to me I listened more intensely than I had in the past as he said, "YOU. "Put both your hand out with your palms up. *God said don't let your left hand know everything your right hand is doing. Which means don't tell everything about you; Keep some things to yourself.*" He warned me, "Listen to me very closely. You have to hear me. Get as close to God as you possibly can. **You are about to lose the most important thing in your life.** You think what I am doing, right here, is something? It is nothing in comparison to what God is going to do with your life. You are going to have a ministry that is going to heal women. You are going to travel the nation speaking a powerful **message of healing**." He didn't stop there, but this time I did.

Immediately, I got it!

How could I ever speak healing to hurting people, if I myself had not been exposed to deep levels of mental and emotional pain?

After all this time, I *still* scramble in failed attempts whenever I try to define the hurt that I felt from my son's death. I finally understand *why*. The pain is indescribable. *I don't know if life offers a pain deeper than the loss of a child.*

AND as if, the burden of Kevin's death wasn't heavy enough, infertility came along and wrapped me like prey in a spider's web. My mind became a playground to heighten levels of vulnerability and insecurity. I wasn't insecure with the image in the mirror, *especially* not after our nutritional lifestyle change. My body had taken on a new form. I had loss *twenty* pounds and I was "*high school fine!*" Yet, I was insecure in my womanhood. Every day, I woke up and went to bed feeling barren because my body wasn't functioning like a woman's body should. I felt in the way of *our dreams* of expand our family. Secretly, I lived in humiliation.

Daily, I had sincere reasons to smile and to be grateful (so I did and I was), but I was lost in laceration. I had drifted so far away from me that I didn't recognize myself any more. My happiness was baseless. My personality was unfamiliar. I tried to embrace the person that I used to be, because I didn't like the person that I had become, but even there I was uncomfortable. The old me was no longer a fit. Mentally and emotionally I was a misfit and this new "*me*" was left devastated, desolated, and totally depleted.

CHAPTER 11

BREAKING OF DAY

After two days of reliving my life I began to write. It was an emotional whirlwind to say the least! The tears burned my eyes like acid. I could barely see my paper, but I stayed consistent. By the end of each night I felt like I had run a marathon. After a week of scripting my anguish, I contacted my friend Jan, an English major, to proof my paper for me. She kindly accepted. A few days later, I received the email with her proofs and I couldn't wait to print and read the draft. As I perused every word, I could not believe what I was reading. *It was my life in black and white.*

As I read, I saw a girl blossom into a woman who I admired. Well, actually I LOVED HER! She was my inspiration! She was strong, resilient, focused and courageous! She was full of consciousness, confidence and determination. She wasn't looking for quick fixes as step by step, she walked out this *struggle* called Life. I could only hope that if sorrow came my way, that I could be as brave as she was. I heard her when she said, "she had reached her breaking point." Now given her track record she just needed to *"create her pause."* She couldn't possibly give up now. She had come too far. I wished that she could see herself through my eyes. *Breaking Point? No way*! I see *The Breaking of Day*! Neither God nor Life could deny her, to do so would be unjust!

After I finished reading MY STORY, I realized it was written it for ME! God had ME to *write it out* so that I could see ME from **A BOLD PERSPECTIVE!**

EVOLUTION

As bright as the light was, before this *very moment* I couldn't see it. I was so blinded by the storms of life. For years I've watched movies, read articles and books (including scriptures), in search for words to permanently remove my pain. The *intensity* remained until now.

As I wrote *("it" out) God erased pain(s). I'm not all healed, at lease not just yet, but the healing process has finally began!* God *is* using *my story* to heal *my life*. As it turns out, my break-through was in my possession. It always was! I just didn't know it.

CHAPTER

12

PROGRESSION

At the top of the 10th month, I went back to the doctor. The first test was an ultrasound to view my fibroids. This ultrasound didn't show it, but at my prior ultrasounds there *were* two pea size fibroids sitting on both sides of my fallopian tubes. Because my doctor thought the fibroids were possibly causing the blockage, I was immediately scheduled for another HSG. When I arrived for the surgery I was notified that because of my doctor's operating schedule she couldn't perform the HSG, and her associate doctor would be performing the procedure instead. When the staff entered the room, the doctor lightened the mood, "So, I hear you love taking HSG's!" I appreciated her humor, but with a grim smile I told her "This is my 4th and final time."

This time, I opted to close my eyes instead of looking at the brightly lit screen. I willed myself not to cry and decided that if my tubes were blocked, I would have a laparoscopy to find out what the problem was. In the midst of my one person conversation, the nurse tapped me with a big smile and gave a thumbs up. I thought it was because I was handling the pain from the procedure, but she looked a little too happy. In the mist of the silence, the next words which came from the doctor still echo a cheerful sound to my soul "YES! This right tube is all the way open. It is over flowing!" Then she said "I can't see the left tube because your uterus is tilted but, you only need one tube to get pregnant!" As the doctor finished the procedure my doctor came in the room with all smiles giving a second "YES! You only need one tube to get pregnant" followed with a high five! To say that it was good news to my ears would be a total understatement!!! Rashon and I left the hospital knowing, without a doubt, that *God's Remedies Work* and we were grateful that He had honored the sacrifice(s)!

FEBRUARY 2014.

In 2012, I started a small business called Sapphire Blue Cake Company. We baked cupcakes for a health conscience clientele. We used an altered version of Grandma Prince's original recipe! Sapphire Blue cupcakes were baked with organic sugar, 50% less sugar than the original recipe along with organic dairy. A few weeks after the 4th HSG, Grandma Prince had a surprise 80th Birthday party. Not only was I on the guest list, but I was also asked to bake the birthday cake and 180 cupcakes.

It was such an honor to be asked to bake for her party because I am part of her legacy!

Four days prior to the party, Atlanta had experienced a severe ice storm; the streets were equivalent to an ice skating rink. Three days prior to the party our Governor declared a state of emergency. Everything was shut down including the airport. My flight was cancelled and rescheduled for the following morning at 7am. I had already lost a day and with so much to do I could not afford to miss my flight. Rashon got me to the airport three hours early. Due to the plane's wings being frozen and the co-pilot being stuck on the highway, we took to the sky an hour and a half late. I asked the flight attendant if I would make my connecting flight. Looking at his pad, he responded "I'm so sorry but your connection has already been changed to 5pm. This flight will land in Minnesota at 10:01 AM. Then the connecting flight to Cleveland takes off at 9:59 AM, and it is scheduled for an on time departure."

In disbelief, I began to silently pray. "God please delay that flight. I can't have a seven hour layover. Aside from not having the patience for such an extended layover, I'm also under pressure because I have to bake and I still have to purchase the majority of my baking items." Suddenly, I was convicted for asking such a thing. A delayed flight was the reason that I was now stuck with a seven hour layover.

The plane landed and I exited the plane at 10:11. I immediately went to an attendant to ask if the flight to Cleveland had departed. I expected the answer to be yes, but I planned to see if there was an earlier connection. I was stunned when he replied, "that flight has been delayed. It is scheduled to depart at 10:19. Run to Gate A6, maybe you can catch it!"

I took off full speed and after a hard push and arriving at an empty gate, I accepted my fate. It was obviously not meant for me to be on that flight! As I stood contemplating my next move, an airline representative came and asked if I needed help. Even though I could clearly see that I had missed the flight, I asked, if the flight to Cleveland had left?" With raised eyebrows followed by a chuckle he asked "Are you Tina Fuller?"

"YES I AM!" I replied.

He responded back "The pilot won't leave and no one knows why." He then asked with intensity "WHO ARE YOU?" The only words that came out of my mouth were "Thank You Jesus!!!" It's *not* about *who I am* but all about "WHO HE IS!" were my thoughts as I hurried down the ramp!

As I stepped foot on the plane the pilot announced "thank you everyone for your patience, now we are free to take off!" As I walked down the aisle, heading toward the two remaining seats, many passengers gave me the evil eye. I took the first available seat on the second to last row, a window seat. After the fight took off my neighboring passenger asked me "Is this your first flight?" Maybe it was my inability to stop smiling or perhaps the way I stared out of the window like a child looking into a candy store. "NO" I replied. I tried to unfold to her what had just happened, even though she showed no excitement.

As I sat in my seat I tried to calm myself, but I had a praise on the inside. God had impressed me! I was full of gratitude and I wanted to yell it from the mountain top, so I went to the little-bitty restroom. I turned on the water and raised my hands, (not to loud because I had already caused a disturbance) and I said, "*God be Glorified!*" I really wanted to shout, you know dance like David did in the bible, but the area was *way too small*. I probably would have burst straight through the little door, so instead I contained myself.

After arriving to our destination, making sure that I was the last person to exit the flight. I went to the pilot and thanked him for waiting for me. He responded "Today is your lucky day!"

I believe that God was showing me not only do I HEAR YOU, but *when you call on me... **I will respond**!*

The morning of the party I was up baking until 5am and grandma was so worth it!

A BOLD PERSPECTIVE

The party was a hit and she was totally surprised! She laughed, cried and danced. Together with family and friends, we celebrated eighty years of life! Everyone marveled over the cake table including Grandma Prince. Before retiring, Mrs. Albertine Prince was one of Cleveland's *baddest (*wedding) cake bakers! Her cakes were delicious and beautiful. To receive a thumbs-up from her (which I did) was a really big deal! But the icing on my cake was the fact *that I didn't leave the party the same way that I came.*

During the festivities, I sat to the right of Chiron. While enjoying myself I saw my cousin Jae coming in the door. I hadn't seen him in about nine years or so, but immediately I was grieved. My mind was swarmed with thoughts like, "Because of you, my son is not here. No way should he have ended up in the street, struck down by a car. In all these years not one Christmas, birthday, Mother's Day or any day in between have you called me to see how I was doing." I couldn't even remember if he ever apologized (but, I'm sure he probably did) and for certain that day in the hospital several stories as to *how* Kevin was hit by the car surfaced. And not to mention, *rumor* had it that Jae and the girl who hit Kevin, were dating prior to the accident.

After being consumed in my thoughts for a while, I found myself telling Chiron my feelings. She responded. "I know this has to be really difficult for you. Jae was headed in this direction but the moment he saw you, his head dropped and he walked to the back of the room."

I asked Chiron to point me in his direction. In the mist of the 200 plus guest, I headed toward him. When I approached him his back was facing me. I gently tapped him on the shoulder and there I stood with open arms. In that moment I broke up with the spirit of unforgiveness.

I forgave him and the entire situation; not because he or they asked me to forgive them... I did it so that we (Me, Him, Kareem and the Girl who hit my son) could be free of *"it"*.

Who am I to hold anyone in condemnation?

Within minutes Jae made his way to the front of the room. He sat at the table to the left of ours. There we were together again, Jamal, Omega, Jae, Chiron and I, were all sitting in close proximity.

During my initial moment of despair, as a pregnant teenage girl while I cried in fear my father held me with *compassion* not condemnation. "We are a family and together we will make it" were his words. So that day, I had my we are a family moment and it was so *liberating*!

HANDS IN THE EARTH

Money doesn't miraculously grow on trees and it certainly doesn't just fall from the sky. Don't get me wrong, I'm not limiting God's power. If He wanted to bless us in that way he could. But instead he chooses to use people to bless people. He uses hands in the earth to convey his blessings.

Give, and it shall be given unto you; good measure, pressed down, and shaken together, and running over, shall men give into your bosom. -Luke 6:38.

As I relive my life, I've realized that my greatest blessings were what I needed the most, *LOVE!*

I am blessed with grandparents, parents, siblings, aunts, uncles, lots of cousins, nieces and nephews. From them I have always received LOVE. It doesn't stop there; I have been blessed with friends, past and present colleagues, clients, church members, class mates, etc... whom have LOVED on me! And when it was time for my next big storm, *Rashon was ushered into my life.*

CHAPTER 13

RE-WRITING THE PAST

*N**ow, with a clear mind...* I know that Kevin was born with a purpose and it is still being fulfilled. I wasn't supposed to see him graduate from kindergarten, fifth, eighth or twelfth grade. *That was never his destiny.*

I also believe that he was supposed to die that day on the bike. In the past, I never understood *why* I was shown that vision...But it had purpose. *Perhaps,* so (someday, [like now]) with assurance I would look back and *know* that his death was meant to be.

I also believe that God wanted to answer my prayers at the hospital, but if He had, it would have ceased my *life's purpose!*

This Journey...This Book... It wouldn't exist without **"The Power of Death."** Kevin, lived and died so that *My Purpose Could Be Fulfilled*!

His death is my *apocalypse.* I have finally *gained* **"GLORY in my BLUES!"**

I hope my story inspires countless lives, but if it only inspires one person to **LIVE** (*in spite of*)...*My Scar(s)* is worth it!

Beauty for ashes, oil of joy for mourning, praise for the spirit of heaviness; **that he might be glorified**. -Isaiah 61:3

A BOLD PERSPECTIVE

OLE GRIEF

Dear Journal March 2014,

Today, I rushed to the computer room prepared to write a new chapter titled Grief, but *mentally* there was nothing there. I had 16 miles (*years*) of grief and I couldn't complete one sentence. The old me would have sat down, focused, and started writing regardless. *This new me* hasn't been the same since seeing my life in print. I am far more refined than I have ever been. I listen to my inner-self. Instead of forcing me to write, I sat quietly. Then a thought occurred, saying "Take a minute and finally listen to the CD that dad sent a few days ago." One Wednesday night he had preached at the mid-week service. I grabbed the CD which was titled, Lord I Just Want To Thank You.

Placing the CD in the player, I closed my eyes and laid back on the sofa. I listened to each word that my father boldly proclaimed. Then he said it "EARTH HAS NO SORROW THAT HEAVEN CAN'T HEAL." I ran and got my notebook and hit rewind. I needed to hear him say it again. "EARTH HAS NO SORROW THAT HEAVEN CAN'T HEAL!" Yeah, I've heard that before, but this time it resonated in the deepest parts of my being! I felt like Jeremiah from the scriptures, the words were like "F-I-R-E!" Instead of in my bones it burned in my soul. It became ever so clear why I couldn't write about grief the way that I had planned too. Spiritually, I had been rerouted!

Since *forgiving*... I hadn't reconsidered my thoughts toward grief. My writing would have been yesterday's sorrow; a false read because I no longer live in yesterday's reality.

Despite opposition, I have had MANY good days, PLENTY of hard days, and thousands in between. Without question, *every day* God gave me strength! Through it *all*, I've been kept sane! I've heard the phrase a million times "He wiped all of my tears away." *Not mine*! Even right now as I am typing, my face is flooded with them! God has allowed me to keep my tears, because they are a weapon; you see, *they purge my heart*. The alkali of my tears have changed from grief to gratitude!

So what do I say to grief?

OLE GRIEF- Let's Cry. Let's Love. Let's Worship. Let's Dance. Let's Laugh. Let's Praise. Let's Live. Let's Forgive and Let's Carry On because our lives and our pain have purpose! HOWEVER, *the* purpose is only revealed on this road called *Journey*. "With every loss there is a gain. *Look for the gain*".

Before I close this chapter, in the words of my father..."Lord! I just want to thank you!

This transformation is *Beautiful!*" After the loss of Kevin, I thought that being *truly* happy was impossible. **I was wrong**!

CHAPTER 14

PERSONAL LIBERATION

There you have it, MY STORY! The one that I didn't want to share... My mind hadn't viewed *"it"* as this.... *My life* has blossomed before my very own eyes!

Yes, God had me to scribe *my story* so that I could see *"the beauty of it"* but it's published for **YOU**...

It's time to HEAL, LIVE, LOVE and FORGIVE!

He shall know the truth, and the truth shall make you free. -John 8:32

Truth is... *The thief cometh to steal, and to kill, and destroy; I am come that they might have life, and that they might have it more abundantly.* -John 10:10

We weren't made to walk around defeated by life's circumstances. When we take on the spirit of defeat, we exalt the adversary by living beneath God's standard for our lives. I was guilty of this. I lived a limited, closed off life because *I made the decision not to forgive.* My life was equivalent to a locked box and until it is opened you can't get anything out of it, and you can't put anything into it. The moment I forgave, I felt an overwhelming sense of peace and instantly I began to love!

I had spent 16 *long* years praying for God to heal my heart. There were times where I thought He had, until Mother's Day, Kevin's birthday, or a movie where a child died would show me that I was still a slave to death's sorrow. At some point I accepted the fact that I would spend the rest of my life emotionally wounded and detached. Then it happened, I let ***"it"*** go and my life took on its own metamorphosis. I emerged from a hungry caterpillar into a stunning butterfly!

Love is (now) filtering healing into my life!

This past Mother's Day was one of the best days that I have ever had! That day was confirmation that I was transformed. Annually since Kevin's passing, Mother's Day *had* proven to be the worst day of my life. For fifteen straight years on that holiday I had a *total meltdown*. "That day" was always filled with pain and confusion. The morning after all the sobbing, I always woke up with my eyes the size of golf balls. Mother's Day 2014 was different because *I was different*. I spent the whole day knowing that at any second I was going to lose it, but I never did!

I opened my eyes *that morning* and looked to my left. Rashon greeted me with such a warming smile, followed by "I've been waiting all morning for you to wake up." As we laid in the bed I tried to quickly assess how I felt. While searching my grey matter Rashon said, "Tina I want to play a song for you." He played "All Of Me", by John Legend, as the song played I dropped a tear, I realized LOVE was all that I felt and I was finally *ready to LOVE* back.

After the song ended Rashon asked me "what would you like to do today?" "Ummm...I want to go to brunch and to the park!" was my response. That's exactly what we did!

We had brunch at Murphy's, a restaurant located in Virginia Highlands; a quaint Atlanta neighborhood. I ordered a waffle topped with fresh strawberries, pan seared salmon and hash browns. As always my experience at Murphy's was delicious! I don't remember what Rashon ordered, but I'm sure it was salmon he's a salmon fanatic. After brunch, we went to Piedmont Park. While there we didn't say much. We walked hand in hand and cherished one another's presence. After walking for quite some time, we found ourselves in front of a landing that is designed for sitting. I stood on it. My 5'2 frame must have become 6'5 as I stood a couple of inches over Rashon. I wrapped my arms around his neck, closed my eyes, and rested my forehead against his. The peace in that moment was miraculous.

"Excuse me. I'm so sorry! I don't mean to interrupt you guys. May I please take a picture? You guys are so beautiful. This moment should be captured!" Spoke a young Asian woman. "Sure! -But only if you take a picture of us with my phone too" I replied.

GLORY AND BLUES

Afterward while walking back to the truck Rashon asked "So what's next Tina?" Well, because I'm a health-nut and I love stores like Trader Joe's, Whole Foods and Farmer's Markets, I asked to go to Trader Joe's. While leaving the parking lot in pursuit of our dinner ingredients, I dropped another tear. Noticing I had a text from my Auntie Chyral, I read these words, "On this Mother's Day, REJOICE in the fact that your child is sitting at the feet of Jesus as he intercedes for all of us. Keep the faith. God is faithful and do know you are so blessed of the Lord!"

On the way home after having a serene and splendid day, I took lots of selfies, as I rode shotgun with my mister. That day is one for the history books!

Wherever I go in life, I will find me. Mother's Day 2014, *I founded a new me because I had changed!*

Prior to Grandma Prince's party, I was stuck in a cycle of unforgiveness, anger, fear, hurt, and even much disappointment. But these emotions could not be brought into submission until I addressed the bigger issue; AVOIDANCE.

No longer could I tote my hurts, in hopes that one day they will just disappear. It was time for me to address *everything* that was afflicting my life, my relationships, and my ability to be free; *mentally, emotionally, spiritually and physically free.*

Side Bar: *If yesterday is gone forever, how long will we remain captive to that which no longer exists?*

No matter what our past and our pain(s) looks like, it is time to deal with it. This journey has shown me, it's not about forgetting, tucking, and running.... It's all about being able to say with acceptance and humility: "***this is my scar***".

In spite of it all...we must develop... so that we may live *life in abundance.* This is no selfish evolution; it can't stop with [self]. It is our *social responsibility* to reach back and grasp others who share a similar pain, frustration, and confusion. *This is how we heal a nation.*

ABSORB THE CALL

Let's imagine our personal homes being a mess. So we've decided to treat ourselves to a house keeping service. After *calling* ABC'S Cleaning Company they have arrived. "*Ding Dong. Ding Dong.*" They are here and ready for the

A BOLD PERSPECTIVE

task. They have all the equipment needed to clean our house, but they can't come in until we *let them in*. Spiritually *"our house"* represents our hearts and our lives. Until we open the door we will remain (internally) *unkept*. Let's *absorb the call!*

We don't all require the same *cleaning detail* because our stories are so uniquely different. My (*major*) detail was avoidance and unforgivingness, yours maybe something else. Nonetheless, IT IS TIME to clean house.

GLORY AND BLUES

WHAT IS YOUR STORY?

Maybe abandonment.

Maybe molestation.

Maybe rape.

Maybe someone you really loved died.

Maybe it's a sickness or a handicap.

Maybe you were wrongfully accused.

Maybe no one ever believed in you or your dreams.

Maybe you grew up in a dysfunctional home.

Maybe you got your heart broken.

Maybe it's substance abuse.

Maybe it's physical or emotional abuse.

Maybe you were the family 'outcast".

Maybe you were bullied.

Maybe it's a generation curse.

Maybe you never felt good enough.

Maybe it's mental illness.

Maybe you did commit the crime, but the suffering was unjust…

Maybe I didn't touch the surface of what happened to you… If so, forgive me.

But the truth is… *it's not my story to tell.*

No one on the plant earth can tell "*Your Story*" better than you.

It is time to *WRITE IT OUT*…

A BOLD PERSPECTIVE

COME! Join me; together let's obtain PERSONAL LIBERATION!

Remember, "Earth has no sorrow that heaven (God) can't heal."

WRITE IT OUT... *Use your journal or the space below.*

PERSONAL CATALOG

For years, I journeyed with a massive cloud: a mixture of negative emotions.

MY CLOUD:

Avoidance. Anger. Hurt. Unforgivingness. Rage. Sorrow. Brokenness. Fear. Pride. Anxiety. Emptiness. Despair. Hostility. Pain. Resentment. Grief. Frustration. Strife. Insecurities.

*Instead of dealing with my cloud, I filled my life with reality blockers: places or addictions where I buried my sorrows or at least **tried too.***

MY REALITY BLOCKERS:

Skating. Shopping. Church. Journaling. Dating. Excessive eating out at restaurants. Schedule-overload. Chick-Flicks. Relocation. Social-Media. Baking Cupcakes.

With every fight, one must have weapons: people or things that leads to victory.

MY WEAPONS:

GOD. Hope. Family. Friends. Laughter. Church. Courage. Dancing. Yoga. Meditation.

Determination. Self-Motivation. Prayer. Goals. Faith.

IT'S YOUR TURN...

MY CLOUD (*Highlight the one[s] that describe your life*).

Anger. Depression. Hate. Guilt. Deception. Bitterness. Jealousy. Unforgivingness. Rage. Violence. Competitiveness. Lust. Insecurities. Sorrow. Brokenness. Fear. Glutting. Sadness. Pride. Self-pity. Doubt. Anxiety. Substance-Abuse. Boredom. Emptiness. Despair. Hostility. Pain. Resentment. Grief. Hopelessness. Death. Blame. Frustration. Impatience. Betrayal. Loneliness. Vulnerability. Sin. Rebellion. Boastfulness. Laziness. Low self-esteem. Strife. Generational-curse.

A BOLD PERSPECTIVE

Lies. Stress. Thoughts of suicide. Etc...

_____

_____

_____

_____

_____

_____

MY REALITY BLOCKERS:

_____

_____

_____

_____

_____

_____

MY WEAPONS:

_____

_____

_____

_____

_____

_____

_____

Let's mold and change our outcome!

WHOEVER or WHATEVER it is that has caused you grief, you must forgive *them/it*.

Not because they asked for forgiveness, but because *YOU can't be bound and free at the same time.*

LET IT GO!

Side Bar: *You may have to forgive yourself. You may have to forgive a person(s). You may have to forgive a system. You may have to forgive God.* I KNOW, forgiving God may sound crazy! But I had too... I felt like God closed his eyes when I needed him the most. *I also asked God to forgive me for being so blinded and so angry.*

A BOLD PERSPECTIVE

I won't make any false promises that right after you acknowledge your issues and *forgive*, that all your hurts will be immediately gone. It is a process, but forgiveness is *powerful weapon* towards your *Personal Liberation*.

MOVING FORWARD

Now that we have addressed our past, *we must guide our futures in the right direction.*

Thoughts of love and positivity about yourself, life and others will promptly change your situation.

For as he thinketh in his heart, so is he. -Proverbs 23:7

Write a list of a dozen positive things that currently describes you or describes the *future* that you desire.

The entire list should written as if it already exists.

- Every line must begin with I AM...
- Place a (F) at the end of the *future* descriptions.
- Make #7 the center of who you are or who you desire to be. (*The number seven represents completion, perfection, security, safety and rest*).
- Make #12 your grand finale. Your finale should be something that, no matter what, *you never waver in.*

MY LIFE

1. I AM NOT A VICTIM TO LIFE OR TO MY PAST!
2. I AM BEAUTIFUL INSIDE AND OUT!
3. I AM STRONG AND POWERFUL!
4. I AM BOLD AND COURAGEOUS!
5. I AM A POSITIVE FORCE OF ENERGY!
6. I AM THE BEST WIFE AND MOM! (F)

7. *I AM A SERVANT OF THE MOST HIGH!*
8. I AM HEALTHY AND WISE!
9. I AM LIVING MY LIFE VICTORIOUSLY!
10. I AM LOVE AND LOVE LOVES ME BACK!
11. I AM FOREVER CHANGED FOR THE BETTER!
12. *I AM NEVER QUITTING ON ME!*

MY LIFE

1. _____

2. _____

3. _____

4. _____

5. _____

6. _____

7.* _____

8. _____

9. _____

10. _____

11. _____

12.* _____

CHAPTER 15

THE RIGHT FUTURE

I have reached a new pivotal point and I have new aspirations!

1. Too much of my life has been spent *trying* to be okay, mentally, emotionally and spiritually. Then fertility challenges brought about physical and financial concerns. I have not only turned the page, but I have closed *that* book. *No more worrying*! From here on out, I will LIVE the rest of my life being in the moment of peace, love, and happiness!

2. I want hundreds of thousands of people to read this book and find their *Personal Liberation*.

3. I want optimum HEALTH, LOVE and WISDOM for me, my family, my friends and every person who reads this book.

4. I want 2 new Fuller babies. Twins please! A son and a daughter for him and for me.

5. I want my husband to fulfill his desires of going back to school. He LOVES education and it loves him.

6. I want to travel the world and experience different cultures through the eyes of the natives. I want to eat, dance, and sing amongst the people.

7. * *I want to be who God created me to be. It would be tragic to miss my life's purpose.*

8. I want a plant-based smoothie bar so that we (The Fuller's) can bring *healing* and *education* to our community.

9. I want to be totally debt free.

10. I want a beautiful "*mortgage free*" home in the Vinings with a finished "*lower level*" for "His" man-cave. Plus a big *sunny* backyard for our garden, a play-yard for the kids, and calisthenics bars for RA.

11. I want a white X6 BMW, but I'll take a white Q5 Audi (*note free too*).

12. * *When it's all over I want to hear the Lord say, "Welcome! Job well done; My Good and Faithful Servant!"*

I hope that you have your journal because it's time to write-out your aspirations!

Same rules apply for #7 and #12.

- Make #7 the center of who you are or who you desire to be.
- Make #12 your grand finale.

Each day that we open our eyes represents a new opportunity to LIVE the life that we desire!

> *For I know the thoughts that I think toward you, saith the Lord, thoughts of peace, and not of evil, to give you an expected end. 12 Then shall ye call upon me, and ye shall go and pray unto me, and I will hearken unto you. 13 And ye shall seek me, and find me, when ye shall search for me with all your heart. 14 And I will be found of you, saith the Lord: and I will turn away your captivity, and I will gather you from all the nations, and from all the places whither I have driven you, saith the Lord; and I will bring you again into the place whence I caused you to be carried away captive.*
> *-Jeremiah 29:11-14*

GOLDEN

Present as today day.
Royal on my throne!
I've been through the fire,
Now, I'm swathed in Gold.

I'm Beautiful.
Look at Me; I AM Beautiful!!
I was Hand Picked.
Broken Into Pieces.
S`H`A`T`T`E`R`E`D!
Then, Molded into My Master's Piece.

The Alter was NO Easy Place,
But ALL for a Sovereign Cause.
I've Been Refined.
I AM Vigorously Present,
I've been REFINED!

Delicate in Character.
But STRONG is my Decree!
The Kingdom Mourns in BOUNDLESS cries,
The Time is NOW!!!
It is Time to Absorb the Call.
All the INSECURITIES,
The Loss. The Pain. That I obtained;
It was All for a *sovereign Cause.*

YES! I WAS Broken.
YES! I WAS Shattered.
But OH!
To be molded by the Master;
It was ALL for a *Sovereign Cause.*
I BECAME STRONG in my Journey!
I AM My Master's Mold!
Look upon ME now; I'M ALL SWATHED in GOLD!
TM.

CHAPTER 16

TEAM FULLER

Within the borders of our marriage, we had been tested emotionally, mentally, physically, financially, and spiritually and in that order. Our marriage started out really good! After our first year anniversary, fertility challenges hit and our marriage went into an emotional spiral. *I* was all over the place and it threw us for a loop.

Currently, we have been in a good space for the past twelve months! In a recent conversation with Rashon, he asked me, "Tina WHY remain good when we can become great?'

In this fifth year of marriage our new marriage goal is to become great!

Q | How has our marriage sustained such turmoil?

1. Spiritually we ***don't waver***. We stood and will forever stand on *"The Rock."* We don't sit down and *wait* for the storms of life to pass over. We are active participants in our outcome. We understand that we must do the work (***fight and develop***), not just for us to conquer and shine in the distance, but to become activists for God's kingdom. Our pain has purpose...

2. Our ***friendship*** *LOVE* allows us to effectively communicate and to support one another. We all know about the emotions of love...and that love is important! *However,* people who love each other get divorced every day. Love is an emotion and emotions change like the weather. The foundation of a relationship has to be strong, not limber. Our friendship love keeps us strong! Despite all the emotions that soar so very high, we always find our way back to our friendship. It is our secure ground; *our foundation*. Spiritually, mentally, emotionally,

physically and financially we genuinely care about each other's well-being. We are dedicated to one another's collective and individual outcome(s). His goals are our goals. My dreams are our dreams.

3. **Communication. Communication. Communication.** *So cliché*, but yet so very true! During the height of the fertility challenges there were so many days where I didn't want to discuss the topic at hand — *my distance, my impulsive dysfunctions*, and things that we could do to improve our marriage. I didn't want to discuss any of it. I wanted to be left alone. I was emotionally ill and each conversation caused such turmoil to an already fragmented psyche. *Hindsight*, I am so glad that Rashon was wise enough to follow the number one bit of advice that we received at our dinner rehearsal party and at our wedding; *communication*! I can still hear Rashon saying, "Ummm Tina, we need to talk!" Never out loud, only in my head, I would say "Damn, again! We need to talk again?" Looking back, I know that I was blessed to have him as a spouse.

4. **Respect.** We respect ourselves and each other! We don't cause blurred lines in our relationship. Blurred lines cause friction and *marriage is tough enough*...

OBEDIENCE

Recently, we were invited to a church service by a family friend, Shonda. One Tuesday afternoon she called. "Hey little sis! You have been on my mind nonstop. I went on a three day fast and prayed for you. After the second day I was so thirsty I told the Lord that I at least needed some water. I didn't get any water, but He gave me strength and I completed the fast! God said that he is about to bless you. He didn't tell me what he was going to do for you, but he told me to tell you that he has a word for you. This weekend my church is traveling from Cleveland to Atlanta. We are having a revival this coming Friday and Saturday. You have to come to either the Friday or the Saturday service."

On that following Saturday after leaving work at 6:37 pm, Rashon and I made our way to the 7 pm service. We took a seat on the back row. At some point during the service the pastor spotted us and asked "Are you guys married?" After we replied "yes", she said, "I need y'all to come up front."

As we were walking towards her, she said, "Oh wow her spirit is so sweet." We stood in front of her with our backs to the congregation as she proclaimed, "I'm not saying the fire is gone, because God didn't say that. However, God is about to fan the flames in this marriage. God said people are watching and If anything happens that causes this marriage not to make it, those watching will lose hope in the institution of marriage." Then she began to tell RA some things about himself. When she got to me she said, "The devil has made a playground out of your mind and it stops today. God said his ears are turned to you, so ask him for whatever it is that you want. God said don't lose your dream, he is going to bring it to past."

Just when I thought she was done speaking to me she said, "Wait! Y'all are trying to have a BABY!"

Then we heard a scream. I turned around to see what was happening, and it was Shonda. She was screaming and running in the opposite direction. During the worship segment of the service as the praise team sang a song using words that proclaimed "GOD IS BREAKING THE CHAINS RIGHT NOW" with a face full of tears Shonda turned to me and asked "Tina- Are y'all trying to get pregnant?"

I answered, "YES!"

She then replied, "God said that next year this time, you will have your baby." So I believe Shonda's screamed in excitement as *confirmation* had come to the words that she had just spoken to me.

After turning back towards Pastor Monique she continued, "GOD SAID THE INFERTILITY IS OVER! He has just sent it back to the sender due to your *OBEDIENCE* and sacrifice!" Then she said, "I need the praying oil. Somebody get it for me. I need to lay hands on these two." She laid one hand on my head and the other hand on Rashon's head. She prayed for both our marriage and my womb. Eventually she had one hand on my head and the other on my stomach as she ministered life to me. In my ear she softly spoke, God said that you are fine. He's been developing you into the person that you are right now!

After service we decided to get something to eat. As routine, after placing my order, I went to the restroom to wash my hands. I looked in the mirror and realized the top of my hair was full of oil. Once I got back to the table I told Rashon she must have had a lot of oil on her hands as she prayed for me. He closed his eyes and shook his head in slow motion and said, "Nah. That's not what happened. She turned the bottle upside down on your head! You didn't feel the oil running?" "NO!" I replied as we laughed!

A BOLD PERSPECTIVE

Then he said, "All I could think to myself was, when she lays hands on Tina after all that oil surely she is going to fall out! Then he followed with I'm surprised you didn't fall out." As I continued to laugh I replied, "No honey, I didn't fall out because my legs didn't give; God needed me to hear and to stand on his word!"

Next I asked him, "So, what will be your first reaction when we find out that we are pregnant?" he smiled and said, "I don't even know."

He returned the question. "I'm not sure either," was my response too.

In silence, I disappeared into my grey matter. I may not know what my first reaction will be, but what I do know is during my entire pregnancy I'm going to praise and worship so much that "The Fuller Baby" is going to come out of the womb with his or her hands up…praising the Lord too! ~AND after I bid my six weeks… I am going to have a David reality….

I was glad when they said unto ME, let us go into the house of the Lord. -Psalms 122:1

The moment I enter the sanctuary to worship, with my husband on my side as he carries our LOVE CHILD! That Day is going to be epic! I might pick up right where little Kevin left off during his last Sunday service. I too will probably shout all the way up the aisle and find myself dancing alongside the drums. At some point maybe the usher will come like Grandpa Lindsey did with Kevin and escort me back to my seat.

Like Kevin I will probably be so full of joy that round two will be inevitable. *This time, LEAVE ME ALONE! When I'm all done,* I'll escort myself back to my seat, thank you! -Bro/Sis Usher *"go and get your own praise on; when praise goes up, blessings come down!"*

I may not know what my original reaction will be… but what I know for certain is I'LL NEVER KNOW, WHAT *DIDN'T* HAPPEN DUE TO DISOBEDIENCE. *God said do it and I got it done!*

Obedience is better than Sacrifice. -1 Samuel 15:22

In the words of Grandma Prince, "*To HELL with the devil.* I'm GOING TO DO *what the Lord said do!*"

Side Bar: *I was at a loss of words after hearing my "saved and sanctified" grandmother say this. I asked her with great concern, "Can YOU say that?" She laughed and said,*

"Yes! Honey, hell is a destination — not a curse word."

The word that came from Pastor Monique on *that night* didn't come until I was almost done writing my story. Fear of self-exposure was laid to rest and faith and obedience wrote this story. When Pastor Monique said that "Don't lose your dream..." It warmed my total being! My dream has always been to be the Best Wife and Mom ever!

THE RIGHT NOW...

With inexplicable patience and genuine love, both God and my husband has chiseled and are mending the broken pieces of my heart. We have not yet conceived, but what we have received is even better. *We got me back!!!* Today I am a better me; an emotionally healthy me! I'm excited about life and love. I am better prepared for when God elevates our family! *I trust the process of love and this beautiful struggle called* LIFE.

OUR story is incomplete... but **that's the BEAUTY of it*!!!*

~ Tina Marie

A BOLD PERSPECTIVE

WHO AM I?

I am a project in its' making!

My past is gone,

My future is yet to come,

My present is here and it is the only moment that I possess.

I Am Life!

In all of creation, there will only be one me;

So I must *make my mark* eternally!

One day, like the wind I'll be gone,

But while here, I didn't *just exist*.

I laughed, cried, danced, sang, worshipped, listened and dreamed.

I fought and *I taught PRO-LIFE!*

I came and *I too*, showed life how to live.

I AM, TINA MARIE, *and this is My Story!*

MAKE IT BEAUTIFUL

Q | In the midst of hurt(s) how do we (The Fuller's) cope with the pains of life?

A | We Worship. We Praise and *We Make it Beautiful!*

Make it beautiful? Yes! Make **"LIFE"** Beautiful! Give back; find a cause, an idea, or a project that you believe in and give of yourself to it.

After Kevin's death I invested myself in ministry. At church I was active on the dance team, new members' ministry and I served as an armor bearer (my pastor's wife personal assistant).

During fertility challenges I started a cake company. It kept my mind occupied. I baked beautiful cupcakes, but after all my research for GOC (section 3), I retired the company.

As a couple, annually we plant a garden with fruit, vegetables, and herbs.

At the forefront of our fertility challenges we created an atmosphere! We decided that we needed something new to receive positive energy from. So, we created an environment that was calming, inspiring, and inviting for professional minded stylists like ourselves and our clients. Into our business model we infused our conscience lifestyle; products without sulfates and parabens.

For us, our Salon was *our Beauty* in the mist of chaos! Even the name *Zero Gravity Concept* Salon, it isn't *just* the name of our business. It's a philosophy, a mindset that enunciates the ideal of breaking free from the gravitational pull and soaring.

Recently, after working all day followed by an evening of cleaning the salon, I looked at RA and said, "It's been two years since we opened and this salon is still beautiful!" He replied "Right now we are standing in our minds. Everything that we see and feel from the music, to the energy, down to the "man-cave" barbershop, it all came from our minds! In essence what you are saying is *we have beautiful minds*!" RA explained.

He *always* has a way of seeing things like only he can!

When life gets tough there is *so much* good that can be done to *MAKE IT BEAUTIFUL!*

A BOLD PERSPECTIVE

One day as a family Rashon, Tashon, Jasrah, Jamal and I we decided to feed the homeless. Together we bagged 50 lunches. Each bag had a sandwich, a juice and cookies. We went downtown and passed them out. *That* inspiration came from a salon client.

A few years back while she was in a TIGHT financial space, one of my clients asked me "Tina if you are available on tomorrow, maybe you and I can feed the homeless. You can bring two loaves of bread and peanut butter and jelly and I will do the same. Together, we can make a bunch of sandwiches and pass them out." That project was one of the host humbling and rewarding experiences of my life. Thx, Tika.

CHAPTER 17

LOVE LETTERS

Dear Chiron and Auntie Jewel~

Thank you for not allowing me to abort my destiny...

Love Tina

Dear Jae and Kareem~

It was meant to be...

P.S. Forgive me for all the years of anger.

Love Tina

Dear Mylon~

I don't know where in life this letter may find you. I haven't seen you in over a decade. I know what Kevin's life did for me, and what his death did to me. But for you, it didn't start or stop there. Life has sent some major blows your way. Before Kevin was born you lost your father. After Kevin died you lost your mother. Some years later, your best friend since childhood passed. *I'm sure there were hurts in between... I am in awe of your strength and your courage to live and to fight another day.*

Our son's life and his death *is* with purpose. I am NOT righting our wrongs... but Kevin was always meant to be. That's how he was so easily conceived... *There's clarity to our mystery!*

*Kevin **loved** you*! At the mere mention that you were coming over to pick him up, his eyes would light up with excitement. Whenever you called to talk to him, he would rush to the phone. As he spoke with you, he would lean against the arm of the sofa (with a *cold lean,* like how you were leaning against *that* locker *that day*... lol). With one leg over the other and with his neck cocked to the right, he would hold the phone with his shoulder and his right hand. Something about him talking to you, even at the age of 2, brought out a cool confidence in him!

Kevin was a strong, fearless kid. Now I see, he was cut from the DNA of both his parents. We just hadn't been through life yet. After all that you have been through, I can hardly wait to see and hear of your *evolution!*

The greater the pain, the greater the progression.

May the peace of God, which passes all understanding, keep your heart and your mind.

Love Kev's mom...

Dear Reader-

Before we continue, I need a favor. May you say a prayer for Kevin's dad?

One close death is more than a notion… Four is way to many.

Call him just that—Kevin's dad. *In real life his name in not Mylon.*

Thank you.

Love TM

Dear Kevin-

A few years shy of a couple decades gone by,

But it still feels like yesterday.

Who would "I" be?

Would I love without fear?

Would the words I LOVE YOU flow without anxiety?

SON, who would you be?

Class clown like your dad or just plain silly like your mom?

I've been trying for such a long time, to put "it" all behind me.

But truth is...

THIS ME? That I am TODAY, doesn't exist without you!

And there is no YOU without me!

Our life together was one beautiful destiny.

Not just our last moment, our EVERY moment(s) was filled with LOVE, hugs and kisses!

Kevin, I would give ALMOST... anything to hear YOU call me again... MOMMY!

But, until that moment, I HAVE A LIFE TO LIVE!

Thanks for changing me 3 times over: *birth, death and now.*

You were such a special child! It wasn't just my life that you changed. You changed the lives of others as well. One year after your death, the daycare center that you belonged to expanded. In your honor, they opened Kevin Lindsey's Preschool Room.

At the ribbon cutting ceremony, the mom of one of your peers spoke. She said, "My daughter was always the subject of bullying. One day, as I entered the day care, I stood watch as a little boy came over to my daughter and snatched her toy away. She said her daughter cried, screamed and hollered. Then a second little boy walked over to her and said, "Stop crying." My daughter proceeded to cry. The little boy who attempted to calm her went over to the first little boy who caused her to cry and he took the toy back and returned it to her. Immediately my daughter stopped crying. Then that same little boy who had just returned the toy to her took it back. My daughter cried even the more. Very calmly he stood there and said, "Don't cry. Ask for it." In a strong voice my daughter yelled, "Give it back!" and he did. As the mom cried, she said "That little boy was Kevin and he taught my daughter how to stand up for herself."

Thank you Kevin for Making It (*LIFE*) BEAUTIFUL!

It was a pleasure being your Mom.

I love you through time and beyond, Mommy

Dear Mom and Dad~

Train up a child in the way he should go: and when he is old, he will not depart from it. - Proverbs 22:6.

Thank you for raising us with a strong spiritual foundation!

Dad, I can still hear you saying "I ain't worried about what other folks are doing in their house. As for me and my house, *We Will Serve The Lord!*"

Mom- I can still here you saying "ask God for whatever it is that you want"! ~AND I can still hear you calling us from way up the street *"KISHA!!! TINA!!! It is time to pray!"*

Side bar: *This was before my parents migrated us to the suburbs. Back then we were in elementary school so of course our friends laughed! Kisha and I stumped and complained all the way back to the house. Once we got inside we already knew there were two choices. You could get your forehead anointed or swallow a teaspoon of the official praying oil - Olive.*

We always took the latter option because going back outside with a shiny forehead was NOT happening! We stood in one circle and prayed as a family. Before the prayer ended Dad would always pray for what sounded liked the "sick and shuddy-end." It wasn't until my adult years that I realized he was saying the 'sick and shut in.' Why he didn't just say those people in hospitals, nursing homes, prisons, etc..? I don't know!

But through guidance and the examples of you guys, in my darkest moments, *I have "lifted up mine eyes unto the hills, from whence cometh my help."* At times the only thing that I had to offer God were my tears, but those tears, they too had to worship. My tears were my expression of worship, because my parents taught me that.

Love Tina aka Tee

Dear Family, Friends, Colleagues, Church Members and Class Mates~

Thank you for ALL the hugs, kisses, smiles, kind words, cards, flowers, prayers, phone calls, time spent, and monetary gifts. Thank you for the investment of love that was deposited into my life. I needed everything that everyone had to offer.

A special *thanks* to my cousin *Tomorrow Dawn Frazier*.

From the moment of Kevin's death until the moment I moved away, you were my eyes and my brain. Through wisdom and love you navigated me. Recently, I had a friend text me and say "Tina my friend and her husband just lost their most precious gift, their seven year old daughter. My friend is in so much pain. What is needed of me?" Tomorrow all I thought about was YOU. I replied to her, "She needs you to love her. Not in the distance, but up close and personal." **LOVE CURES INSANITY!** What you became for me, is the advice that I gave to her.

Kevin Frazier, thanks for allowing me to steal your wife. I needed her presence like air. For *years* she and I spent HOURS hanging out at the mall, restaurants and talking on the phone and you allowed it...

To my cousin **Tammy**, I remember the car rides too... thank you!

Love Tina

Dear Rashon~

Please pardon me, as I lack the words to express my sentiment. Perhaps, if possible we could switch hearts for just a few minutes, then maybe you could scribe the perspicacity of my affection. It's *so deep* that one would almost have to be Elocutionist to do so.

Much LOVE and GRATITUDE, Teen

ALMOST DONE...

Yes everything in section one is true. Not one detail did I make up (except some names). I didn't have too. With my *hands out and palms up*... I left out plenty of details...

Mister in the clergy collar... You don't know who I am, but I do know who you are!

One day while at school (high school) at a distance amongst hundreds of students scrambling the halls to get to our next class, I saw you. You were with one of my classmates. You're the dad of one of my tiger nation peers! One day *soon* I will pay you a visit. I owe you a big hug! *That day* God sent you on a mission to deliver a word to me. Until we meet face to face for the second time, thank you Sir for your *obedience*!

Before we turn the next section over to Rashon, *Grandma Prince has something that she would like to say...*

-By the way, Rashon and I chose not to read one another's writing until the book is release. So, I can hardly wait to read section two!

GRANDMA PRINCE...

I could see by the caller ID, that it was Grandma, so I answered, "Hey Grandma!"

She replied, "Hey my beautiful! How are you feeling today? How is everything going with your book?"

I replied, "I am doing good and the book is going better than I ever expected. I am working on the last chapter as we speak!"

Then she said, "That's wonderful Tina! I know that you are a busy lady so I'm not going to keep you on this phone, but I want to know, in the book are you going to have a picture of me and the family?"

"Ummmm... I hadn't planned on having any pictures of the family" I replied.

"Oh okay I was just wondering," as she followed with, "Well one more thing. You pray about it first, but I believe that in your book you should share what

GLORY AND BLUES

God showed me"...

All because you asked, it is so... xo

"We have a very close family and everybody absorbed the pain of Kevin's death. Deep grief was upon everyone. Of course no one was more hurt than, my Tina. We were all hurting and I didn't have anyone to talk to because I didn't want to make anyone hurt any more than they were already hurting. Every day the entire family gathered to comfort Tina. About a week or so after his death I came home tired and overwhelmed with grief. I had lost my great grandson and the hurt that my granddaughter was experiencing was too much to bear.

One day after coming home from Reynold and Val's house (Tina's parents) with a heavy heart, I laid back on my green leather sofa. I was *not* asleep, my eyes were opened and God took me off into a vision. *There Kevin stood dressed to perfection like a king's kid. His body language was like that of a man, but he was still a kid. He stood before the Lord and gave his account of you. [Oh Tina, I wish that you could have seen him!] He was beautiful! In this vision I could only see the feet of God, but I saw Kevin in completion. I will never forget the tone of Kevin's voice as he spoke so very proper and clear.* "MY MOTHER TINA, WAS A GOOD MOTHER! SHE WAS PATIENT AND KIND!" *It was almost like he spoke in a question form, as if to say, now God WHY would you take me away from a mother like that?"*

She continued "Tina, God has the record! Kevin gave a good report of you! *All parents* need to understand that their children will stand before the Lord and give an account for or against them. *Love your children and do what's right by them."*

LOVE, *Grandma Prince*

A BOLD PERSPECTIVE

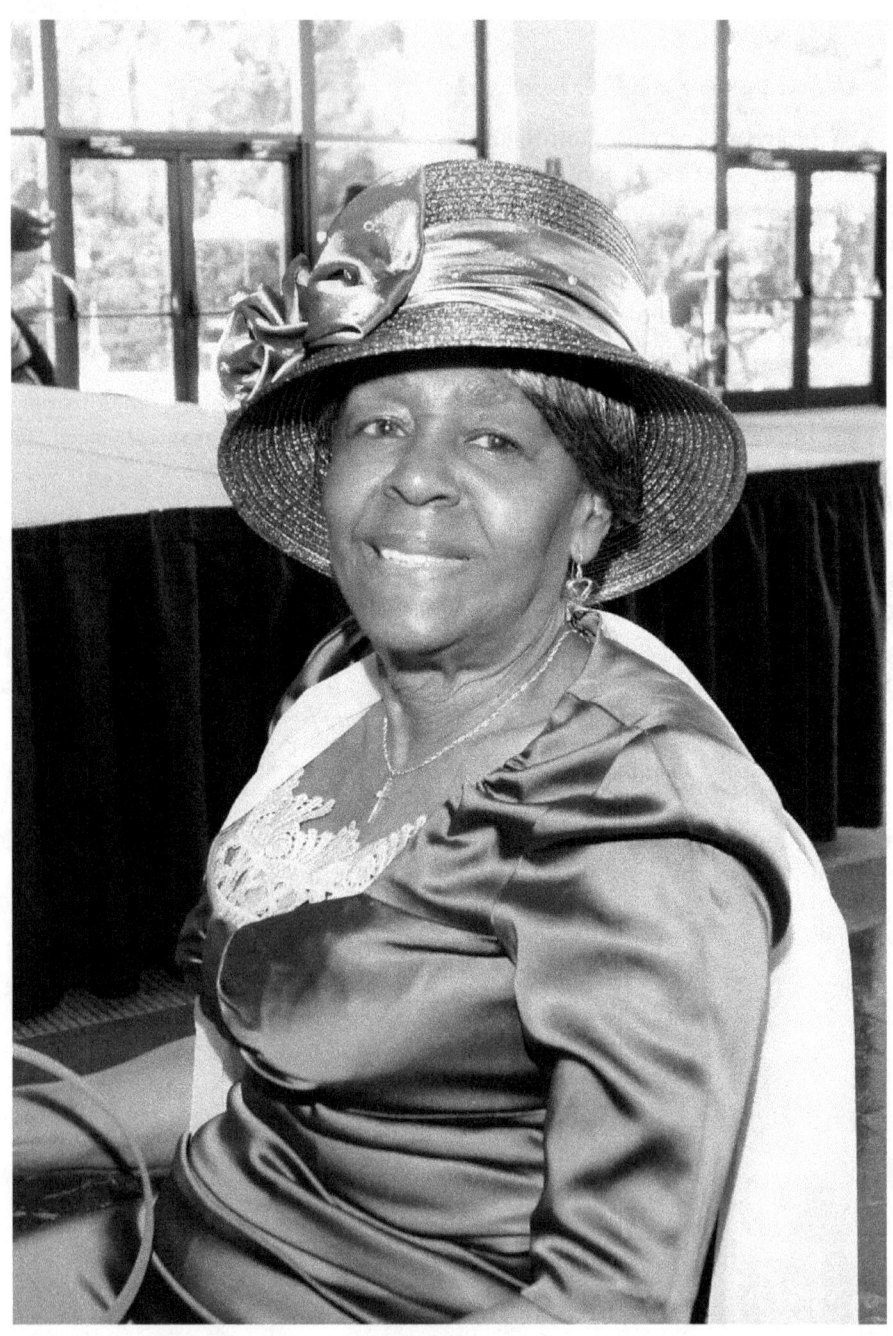

SECTION 2
LIFE IN ABUNDANCE

INTRODUCTION

The reality is everyone has a story and an intrinsic desire to express it to others. The estimated total population of planet earth is approximately 7 billion. The population density, which is people per square mile, is 105 globally.

So many of us seem to get lost in this giant sea of people, finding it all but impossible to comprehend why our personal stories are so unique. We may constantly lose sight of just how special we are, and the extreme rarity we possess. Just like no two fingerprints are identical, the same holds true for each individual's human experience. It's like macro versus micro and how it relates to the human cells. Identical twins share many characteristics, but their experiences will certainly differ.

The old saying, "We are the sum of our life's experiences" certainly holds true for each individual. These experiences leave indelible impressions on our lives and become the catalyst for how we function. I believe there is a magic in every story which heals, inspires, motivates, educates, prevents, and delivers while breaking chains and providing justice in some instances. Although the human experience happens to us, we still have the innate ability to create our own thought patterns and behaviors, make our own choices, and chart our own course in life.

Every human being is made of the same material that we find in the universe. It is the awesome design of these atoms infused with consciousness within that makes it even more complex. It is not just matter but thinking matter. The popular belief that the quickest way to the center of the universe is up or outward is false. Fact is, going within either mentally, spiritually, or physically would be closer to being mathematically correct. In ancient eastern traditions this act of going within to pursue knowledge of self is considered the path of enlightenment. Each atom that makes up our physical composition is connected to the entire Universe. By studying the Microcosm we begin to understand the microcosm "as above so below" a thorough study of the seen often exposes the reality of the unseen.

As a basketball fan, I've always been in awe of Michael Jordan's story. He was an amazing all-around athlete... six time NBA champion, trailblazer known for game shots at the final buzzer, franchise owner of a NBA team, and brand ambassador for Nike the most profitable athletic apparel company. However, the most amazing part of Mr. Jordan's story is the part when he was cut in the 11th grade from his high school basketball team. Wow…the greatest basketball player of all time was once told he wasn't good enough. Imagine the transformational process he went through the summer before his senior year. Michael Jordan made the choice to condition and train, and he showed up for his senior year in a zone. Not only did he have a phenomenal year, but he secured a full ride to The University of North Carolina!

Due to the reality that we are only here for a relatively short time (120 years or so), we are able to hack life by studying history and the stories of others to extract precious jewels for our personal development. Albeit, all stories have positive and negative elements we still benefit from.

There are some stories that speak to us more than others. This is just a fact of life. However, I believe with my whole heart that this is a story that anyone who has breath can connect to. This story is about complete transformation and healing.

I have been blessed to witness an incredible transformation right before my own eyes.

There is a feeling of redemption when watching someone you love go to their lowest psychological, emotional, and mental depth then recover. I'm not speaking of a bad day or a tough week. No, I'm referring to a psychological trauma so severe that not even the universal healer we know as time could remedy the brokenness. This trauma was heavy, dark, and engrained in the heart of my loved one. I have experienced going from sharing a full throated laugh to unstoppable tears within one real life picture frame. This experience for me was raw and unyielding, yet it was the authentic human experience. This was a pain so intense, one had to navigate through the mind's saturated landscape of general conversation with adroitness, because one wrong word, or incorrect reference could prove costly. In front of me was a tortured soul and all I could do was pour love into this vessel. It was a genuine and unconditional love, with the understanding that reciprocity was possibly not an option.

To see the mercy of God come forth and heal what seemed unable to be restored was nothing short of a miracle. I watched Him provide beautiful clarity of mind where there was once complete confusion. I witnessed POWER and

GRACE where there was once weakness and doubt. Clairvoyance replaced the permeating question of, "Why me?" Purpose driven days took the place of aimless agendas, where happiness, faith, love, and hope were all restored right before my eyes.

I'm speaking of the woman who I firmly believe was designed for me, Tina Marie Fuller. After losing her son, Kevin, I've personally witnessed this incredible and amazing soul rise from the ashes like the mythological creature known as The Phoenix Bird, adorned with resilience and fortitude. The two of us have been on a journey together. We've made lifestyle changes for a better quality of life and spiritual connection with one another. So, when she asked me to contribute to this assignment she received from the Most High God, it was imperative that I lend my voice to this project. It was a no-brainer! I am so proud of my wife for her courage and ability to tell her story of despair and triumph (after the loss of her son) to the world and expose her naked truth with the hope of touching others. There is something redeeming about this experience for me. As a father, I find myself pondering if I could stand as boldly as Tina if I lost one of my offspring. I hope to never experience that, but at the same time I feel so deeply her emotions for the loss of her baby. Perhaps it's our covenant that has me so connected to her experience because our paths did not cross until after her loss. I've personally experienced an array of emotions with her, though not on the level that she feels it. Like a powerful architect I see God's hand building, and shaping his concern. Through all of this, I am reminded that HE is REAL.

CHAPTER 1

POWER OF LOVE

Every since I was a little boy, I wanted to be in love. Love was all around me. I experienced it in some of my favorite movies. In fact, I find it difficult to remember any movies back then that didn't have a love story in its theme. I also discovered this magical force in music, as well. Although the complexity of the lyrics would elude me, until the maturation of Rashon would occur. I still felt its power.

Then there was the third grade crush, Dana. That day started very normal in class. We were working in groups on a project. I was counting down the time, until recess and daydreaming about playing four square and two hand touch football with my friends. Then I heard our teacher say, "Class, may I have your attention? I would like you to welcome our new student, Dana."

All of a sudden the day wasn't normal anymore. Trumpets blared in the background and the air was full of the scent of cherry lip gloss. I think it was safe to say, I was struck without warning. Then to add fuel to the fire, our teacher Mrs. White said, "Mr. Fuller, stand up please."

I could feel myself take a big gulp as I stood to my feet.

She then said, "Could you be so kind as to be Dana's partner for the day? Please introduce her to the rest of the class and help her get settled in."

As history would have it, Dana became my first girlfriend. My early learning experiences on love are so special because I didn't gain them in the obvious places like watching my parents. Unfortunately, romantic love didn't exist between my parents. It wasn't something I experienced.

A BOLD PERSPECTIVE

My mother and father were divorced by the time I was three. I've never seen my parents kiss, embrace, or hold hands. I do not have a single memory of hearing my father tell my mother "I love you," like I saw in all the movies I watched growing up. Sadly what I experienced was a dysfunctional relationship on both sides.

Yet, instead of being jaded by love, I desperately wanted it. It had the opposite effect. I yearned to find that special woman with whom I could engage and connect with.

Without a model of what love and marriage look like, it was certainly a matter of trial and error for me. After a few failed attempts and close misses, I was able to discern the reality that it simply requires the right mate to pour your love into in order to receive that love back. It's more than good looks and exterior qualities that dictate the love experience.

There was a point in my life in which I had given up on love. I began to subscribe to the belief that love is a game, and I coupled that with the psychological residue left over from my dysfunctional upbringing. But then, one day the stars aligned and the visual of the sad lady in the purple dress who lulled me with her divine spirituals stopped….mid-verse. The image simply dissipated because my wife entered my life!

For the first time ever, I knew I had gotten it right. I loved her and I believed, without a shadow of a doubt, she loved me back. After all of the praying and dreaming, I finally found her. "Swing wide the gates, and let the trumpets blow!"

Everything was perfect. It was like a dream come true. Now I could finally relate to the type of love that was being sung about in my favorite reggae tunes. Tina was from a good family and was raised with sound biblical principles. We communicated well about everything. Our conversations were about family, our future, personal goals, diet, education, and many other things. There was a depth and understanding that the two of us explored in every conversation and it provided an assurance for me.

Like all marriages, we had disagreements but within boundaries and always out of respect. The foundation was on a square and we were equally yoked. Our union was indicative of what most deem a fairytale. There were long walks in the park holding hands, "chopping it up" about any and everything. No topic was off limits because we were a safe place for each other. Our personal and business lives were ultimately weaved into one, and we were inseparable!

I remember driving home one day and thinking to myself, "Someone, please pinch me because this is too good to be true." Life was good!

This euphoric feeling was challenged after about six months into our marriage. A disconnection was noticeable and I was blindsided. Intimacy and affection was fading and it was happening fast. I could tell my wife was shielding herself from something, and that something was ME. I had an idea of what the source was which helped me to cope somewhat, but my touch and kisses were met with resistance, and frustration was certainly becoming a constant companion. I began to relate to the unlucky guy who slips into the friendship zone with a person he loves so deeply. Unrequited love slowly tried to creep into our union, and I battled with the emotional void that seemed to accompany intimacy. We had evolved from friends to lover, and here we were again back at "friend." This wasn't what marriage was supposed to be. Instead, marriage was to represent the universal language of love...AGAPE love, to be exact. The love of altruism which is giving without asking anything in return, and of sacrificing oneself for one's partner. Many would consider it to be the purest form of love. Most couples, regardless of the culture, can relate to this type of love. The phrase "I Love You" should require no explanation in a marriage- only action. Yet, there were limited actions being reciprocated by my wife that resembled love.

My world was shaken and harsh realizations flooded my thoughts. It was like being blindsided. Our courtship had informed me otherwise and I thought we were going to be the model couple. The truth was, my wife had emotional barriers that were really no fault of her own. Her loss had altered the course of her life in such a major way and she was operating with a fragile psyche. A sobering reality began to settle in and sadness consumed me. I knew for sure that I loved Tina with every fiber in my body. So I mustered up all of my emotional fortitude and I confronted my wife.

I vividly remember the day I approached Tina. I was sure to take my time to lovingly and eloquently explain my feelings. She listened carefully to what I had to say without any interruptions and even gave an occasional nod of agreement. Once I had shared my heart with her, she gathered herself and shared her honest response which was surprising to me. She actually validated everything I had been feeling and explained that she was very aware of our intimacy issues. She explained that it was of no fault of mine, but was related to the death of her son. Her words are still etched in my mind.

"After experiencing this kind of loss, the reality of letting my guard down and loving new people doesn't come easy. I even find it difficult to tell my own mother and father that I love them."

Although I empathetically understood her position, it left me in an awkward position. I pondered how to love her past her pain and move forward. Did this mean that I would experience my wife in a guarded and shielded way? Would reciprocity ever be an option?

I experienced my "aha" moment where a plan was very clear. If I gave it everything I got and poured my unconditional and unyielding love into my wife, I could break down the walls she had built. I was determined to show her what real love could feel like. My actions would allow her to see that LOVE does not have to hurt. Instead, it could heal and restore what was broken.

Victory was the goal as I steadied myself to execute this strategy to win my wife's affection. I put it in fifth gear. I knew what we had was too special to not fight for it. Over time things began to improve. Bob Marley's music was the soundtrack to my life: "Don't worry about a thing, cause every little thing is gonna be alright!" I was persistent and sure enough things were on an upswing. I put in the work and she responded in love.

Then we decided it was time to add to our family. We wanted to hear some little footsteps around the house. We were extremely excited about the idea of having a child together. We were very aware of the impact this would have on our relationship, but we began the process for conception. We had established a connection and were on one accord about everything that this step entailed. But, I honestly was unaware that another emotional shift was about to happen. Sex became very regimented and lacked romance. It was about HAVING A BABY!

After a significant amount of time and numerous tries, we didn't conceive. I sensed her anxiety and it became evident that we had a new challenge. Frankly, I was completely blindsided by the challenges brought on by infertility and so was Tina. Temperature checks, ovulation dates, and scheduling replaced the passion that used to accompany lovemaking. I've always been keenly aware of the consequences associated with a lack of birth control. This is the type of banter that happens every day in barber shops all over America. Man Code, so to speak. It's certainly what men talk about when they are amongst themselves.

However, I have no recollection of discussing infertility in any arena. In retrospect, I understand it's usually not something that most people feel comfortable talking about. It certainly was not something I had considered for myself.

Initially, our inability to conceive was hard for me to come to terms with. My thoughts kept gravitating to "any day now we will conceive." In the beginning, we both were patient with the process. But eventually, awareness and raw emotions surfaced.

In this life there are certain events, moments of time that stand out in our minds fresh like they just occurred yesterday. For me, my wife asking me how I felt about going to the doctor to get examined for infertility challenges was one of those moments.

"What! You want me to get checked out. This thing is going too far!" My reaction was scathing but genuine.

On the surface I appeared irritable and agitated at the mere request. "There is nothing wrong with me. This is a huge waste of time! I know everything is working fine for me. This is pointless and demeaning," I retorted.

My wife was persistent, to say the least. She calmly (well maybe not so calmly) said, "My doctor has requested that you get fully examined before we go any further with my test and examination. We must eliminate you as an option, and then proceed."

There was a clear distinction between my response and my inner thoughts which were laced with fear. "What if it is me?" "How will it affect our marriage?" "As a man if I am unable to procreate, how will that define me?"

I began to think about how humiliating it would be when I'm asked, "When are you and Tina going to have a baby?" I thought, "How will my wife view me moving forward, if the issue lies with me?" Looking in her eyes and seeing her resolve forced me to confront my fears. I said, "Ok I will go."

That day came and I was very nervous. I'm generally a private person outside of close friends and family, but when I showed up to the fertility doctor's office everyone seemed to know exactly why I was there.

A woman in her early twenties gave me instructions and showed me to a room. She handed me some magazines and before closing the door, I could have sworn I saw a smirk on her face. Maybe it was just my imagination, but I decided to get it over with. I began to notice just how deeply all of this was affecting my wife. She slipped back into an unhealthy place. To say intimacy was once again affected would be an understatement. It was as though all the love and affection had been sucked out of the relationship. Simple expressions of love like a hug or a kiss became painfully awkward.

I was on egg shells while waiting on the results of the test. Meanwhile, back at the ranch the "infertility behemoth" was wreaking havoc on our day to day lives. It was like a continuous nightmare.

One day we were doing fine watching a movie together until a pregnant lady appeared on the screen. Just like that, the mood shifted. It was evident the emotions were just too raw to deal with rationally.

When my results finally arrived, everything was good on my end which was a relief. I'm not sure how I would have felt; if I had found out I was infertile. Relief quickly turned into concern. In hindsight, I see why the emotions I experienced were so important. It prepared me to understand some of the emotions my wife would be up against.

The challenges of infertility are a heavy burden for anyone to carry. To add a traumatic loss to that equation is enough to tip the scale. I made a decision to love my wife through it all.

I would kiss her until the kisses were returned.

I decided I would never allow a finite situation or unchecked energy define us and determine our faith. This battle called for the full armor of God moving forward. As a student of life, I have learned the importance of being humble and open to receive the lesson.

I thought, "God is at the helm steering the ship to the shores of our destiny, although we don't know when we will be with child. But we know what his/her name will be, and we also know our baby will be loved beyond measure. We will work to ground him in faith and the Word of God. For now that's sufficient for us. Our faith, our dreams, our powerful imagination, and hope are what we have to move forward. What we focus on most is where our power lies. In reality, that's all we can control."

Now that we have experienced the challenges that came with infertility, there was an extra sensitivity shown towards others dealing with a similar circumstance. We knew that together we were confident that all of this had a divine purpose and it would somehow lead us to our path.

CHAPTER

2

GENESIS

"In the beginning God created the heavens and the earth."

This is the magnificent way the Bible begins. With no delay we are immediately introduced to the mighty God. We learn that He is the architect of the heavens and the earth. If all the oceans were flowing with ink, it would run dry if I started to pen the magnitude of that verse! Suffice it to say its power never fails to blow my mind. I have really given this some thought. There is no question that the earth is massive and glorious in its design. It is full of wonder and undiscovered secrets. A mere attempt to take in all the earth's wonder would have one's eyes suffering with endless fatigue. Now this heaven part is so heavy I find myself having to close my eyes and just meditate on the magnitude of the reality, a universe known to be infinite in size. What this opening verse is saying is this mighty God created the entire universe from nothing. Talk about setting the bar high.

Next, the Bible elegantly begins to explain what was created over the next seven days. Something special happened on the sixth day. Genesis 1:26 says, "and God said, Let us make man in our image, after our likeness: and let them have dominion over the fish of the sea, and over the fowl of the air, and over the cattle, and over all the earth and over every creeping thing that creepeth upon the earth."

This is the secret of all achievement revealed in this 26th verse. We have already been introduced to the omnipotent creator and His majestic creation. Now He gets around on this sixth day to creating man. Unlike all the other creations, as marvelous as they were, they were not created in God's image or after His likeness as man was.

This gives us the blueprint of our purpose and power. Our Father, who art in heaven, gave us a piece of His mind and a portion of His power. After GOD made man, He gave him very strict instructions to justify his existence. This beneficent LORD made it plain that all He created was made to be subdued by man. Being fruitful and multiplying was a direct instruction. When we conceive a ideal we have the awesome power like our Father who art in heaven to manifest that ideal, and bring it forth. Yet unlike GOD who creates from nothing, man has all the material he needs to clothe the ideal already in the earth!

In this world, we often find ourselves with feelings of inadequacy, having low self-esteem, doubt, and even pessimistic thoughts. Our minds have been shaped by various institutions that are insufficient to guide what they didn't create, form, or fashion.

Capitalism, for example, is a system here in America that we operate under. It requires conformity of education: training in a sense that corporate droning begins in the schools where students' independence and creativity is driven out of them. We often find ourselves in a world we don't really understand and a reality we are ill equipped for. These institutions that shape the minds of man have defined motives for their curriculum. It is simply to feed the machine workers. This is why I personally find so much solace in the scriptures.

The seemingly powerful elite in this world who sit in positions of high status function as megalomaniacs. This elite group is obsessed with their sense of power over others dragooning the masses into their conspiratorial subterfuges. This condition leaves many precious human beings laboring to carry out determined ideals that have no connection to their divine purpose. I feel the need to touch on this condition to highlight the majesty of the one Most High God! Genesis helps us understand God is not just omnipotent. He is also gracious enough to be in the power sharing business, unlike the above stated megalomaniacs. We have been commissioned with His power to do His will. To be unaware of our power is like forfeiting our purpose in this life. The ideal of Genesis lends one's thinking to change or the redemptive quality that allows us to start new.

One of the greatest forms of study, I have found, is the study of our self. There are so many levels to peel back. What I have found is the world around us is essentially a macrocosm and the world within is indeed a microcosm. With a thorough mastery of self we can bend the circumstances of life around us to our will.

LIFE IN ABUNDANCE

What are you waiting for to change your reality? Ok, so life dealt you a tough hand. Maybe the adults around you, trusted with your safeguard, failed majorly. This is a painful reality that has the ability to position the self-proclaimed victim into a perpetual state of melancholy.

However, the good news is there is a cure from this dreaded condition. We are participants in this activity. We know life is equipped with the ability to shape our reality after our thoughts. Of course, this design works just as well for both positive and negative thoughts. If your thoughts are of the reoccurring negative type, that has its origin in the past. Then that is what you will create. You will mold the world outside of yourself to resemble the thoughts you're entertaining on the inside of your mind.

Now if we can make a practice of loading positive thoughts into our mind, then our lives will take on the reality of those thoughts. There is a tremendous amount of power in a negative as mathematics teaches us. For example: $-1 \times 500 = -500$; one negative has the ability to change the charge of 500 positive potentials.

There is nothing as sad as unattained human potential. We are commissioned by the Almighty to discover, uncover, and deliver our gifts given to us.

CHAPTER 3

CREATE YOUR PAUSE

One day I was driving down the street and had a thought. "What if I could pause all the circumstances around me and give myself a clear unobstructed path to my goals?" I mean the bills, personal issues, eliminate the pressure of all those deeply depending on me, etc., and just put it all on pause. Then I laughed out loud at the weakness of the thought. Who ever achieved anything great by pausing all the many factors of life to do so?

Okay, if by some stroke of magic we could do this, would we even consider it to be great? Life is indeed a gift, but it comes with a design. Better yet, I should say it comes with the ability to be designed. The way our life is set up is usually the result of multiple events, creating an outlook and a pattern that we follow robotically fearing the perceived consequences of breaking the pattern.

There is awesome raw power in a painter staring at a blank canvas, a writer staring down a blank page, or a songwriter with an instrumental beat. That powerful moment, right before the art gets created, can be intimidating for the artist.

Every day when we rise, the day is new and equivalent to a blank canvas. We can create and design the new day to our imagination. The initial spark is usually the most difficult part of the process. There is often a blank in terms of what direction to take the creation. There is the flood of thoughts in no particular order that comes with the process. This can be confusing. It often causes one to quit the potential creation.

The irony is right after that sometimes difficult beginning, the thoughts begin to heat up a flow allowing the creator to construct the creation. This is a process so beautiful; it makes the soul feel like a flower in bloom. This activity we call life can be designed and molded to create the reality that one would call their lifestyle.

If you don't take the bull by the horns, then life will blow one circumstance after the next like the wind in your life. Now that you didn't take the offensive, circumstances now delegate your moves. Many of us find ourselves in this holding pattern in our lives hoping, wishing, and praying from life's unrelenting pressures. Thinking in this pause, we will find the energy, ideas, and resources to be great.

This simply is not the case. The chaos we experience in our daily lives is simply just a manifestation of our thoughts. From my vantage point, the obsession people seem to have with celebrities is that they appear to buck the natural order of things. The illusion is that these celebrities live in this fantasy like worlds where they completely unfold their gifts, talents, and purpose, which seem to elude so many. Even their trials and tribulations appear poetic; the essence of the phrase "the truth appears stranger than truth."

When we speak and think of freedom, oftentimes it's about no restraints, coming and going as we see fit, able to make our own choices, and the resources to finance our ideals. In reality, those definitions ring true, but I would venture to say there are many IED's on this path. The noise is deafening and the distractions are many. So often, we truly discover freedom once the ideal of freedom we have is taken away.

If a visit to the doctor reveals a discovery of cancer, then instantly we begin to reexamine our lives combing through priorities. This tends to break the pattern (at least temporarily) of how we move and think. We can also add to this list prison, loss of life, loss of money/job, relationship issues, witnessing the terrible human suffering and many other things. I once heard it said, "A man who is robbed of patriotism is robbed of a good thing."

As part of the human experience, we tend to find meaning in groups we belong to or associate with. For example: teams, family, school, fraternities, organizations, religious groups, cities, states, nations. In order to fully reap the benefits one must start with a thorough knowledge of one's self.

CHAPTER

4

INSTAGRAM VS. REALITY

"A picture is worth a thousand words."

My father once said to me in his I'm-about-to-drop-some-jewels-of-wisdom-voice,' "Son if you live to be 90 years old and you can count your true friends on one hand, you did damn good." Well Dad, your wisdom may have reached an expiration date, because here I am, nowhere near that age and already I currently have over 6,000 friends.

Well, that is if you add my Facebook, Instagram, and Twitter accounts together. The reality is that we live in a burlesque of social media. Feelings of being weird, friendless, isolated, and alone are no longer in vogue thanks to these incredibly ingenious social platforms.

Well, hang on a minute, not so fast. Designers conceived in Instagram a unique concept of delivering content rapidly in the form of photos. These photos are intended to represent your lifestyle. If the metaphor a picture paints a thousand words holds true, then the photo for content design packs a mean punch! When you scroll down your timeline, you see all the personalities posting the latest event to unfold in their lives. You know they are hoping for a healthy applause communicated through double taps. On IG, ones social status is directly associated with the amount of followers and likes that are received. The culture seems to rank those who post fresh content and receive a few amounts of likes low on the social hierarchy.

This seriously damages the ego, suggesting one's life content is either not interesting or not important. Instagram, as well as other social media apps, has

A BOLD PERSPECTIVE

in many ways become a measuring stick for one's popularity. It is a judgment of how 'turned up' a person's day to day lifestyle is. We put our lives out there to be judged and wait anxiously for approval. It's not unusual to see people checking their pages via smart phones every few minutes throughout the day, religiously.

CHAPTER

5

THE SELFIE

If a tree falls in the forest and there is no one to hear it, does it make a sound? Or perhaps the modern equivalent is, if someone has an experience without taking a selfie, did the experience actually occur? How did one's own picture ever become so Omni-important?

The emergence of The Selfie is pure narcissism. I wonder if Steve Jobs had this in mind when he decided on the catchy name of iPhone, iMac, iPod, etc. Did he know people would become islands submerged in a state of subjectiveness? There is simply not enough real touch interaction in my opinion, and I can only wonder how this is ultimately affecting the world.

When did creating the illusion that one's life is awe-inspiring supplant the necessity of creating an awesome reality? One of the most powerful activities we can engage in is experiencing the moment with all senses engaged.

A few months ago, I met one of my favorite artists, Rakim. Thanks to a mutual friend, I was able spend an hour backstage with him. As rich as this moment was for me, at no point did I make the toxic mistake of pulling out the camera and turning the moment into an Instagram alert. Instead, I totally embraced the experience. Talking very little, but observing and taking it all in. It was not only one of those cherished moments that I will always value, but I believe the exchange was mutually received as well.

The reality is social media is a brilliant innovation. When used effectively as a tool, it can be an asset to network, build and market businesses, and leverage as a platform for connections. What it doesn't do is replace the human need for face to face interaction with touch and smell. I urge you all. Forgo posting your

A BOLD PERSPECTIVE

life for a while and just experience it instead. Embrace mindfulness. You don't need a photo to create a memory. You don't need others to believe it happened. Just Be There.

CHAPTER 6

THE BEAUTIFUL STRUGGLE

I know what you're thinking. There is no beauty in struggle right? I believe one of the greatest impediments to our success is the inability to see the struggle in the proper light. According to divine scripture, struggle is ordained for all of creation. There is a struggle involved for the sperm cell to reach the egg. The sperm must travel through a very hostile environment, although millions of sperm cells are released, but typically only one will reach the designed destination. So we are engaged in a struggle from our very beginning.

One winter evening, I was relaxing with my wife lying in front of our fireplace. As the wood burned, I found myself in a deep trance like meditation. My eyes were drinking in all the amazing activity that was taking place. A combination of combustion, snapping, and crackling gave birth to an array of colors exploding like a well-choreographed dance. Wood has a thick skin with heavy moisture made to repel the intense inferno and slowly release heat as its body returns to the essence.

As beautiful as the fire was, the light that was thrown off could not provide my skin with the vitamin D it needed to be radiant, nor could plants complete their photosynthesis process from the light of a wood fire. Fire that uses wood as fuel is impotent in comparison to the giant magnetic ball of fire located approximately 93 million miles away from the earth known as the sun. This huge ball of fire emits an altogether different light that has life giving properties within it. The difference being the cause of its combustion is ignited by a divine magical source. The power if this magical fire is that it is able to burn away the impurities of a thing stripping it down to its essence.

A BOLD PERSPECTIVE

When we see a blacksmith apply fire to steel, it then allows him to mold and shape the substance to his will. I have arrived at a somewhat unique perspective concerning the reality of the struggle. There is no living organism under the Sun that is exempt from the struggle. Life itself is a struggle. Even with the most abundant love we cannot shield our cherished loved ones from struggle. It is struggle, not ease that shapes and develops us. Quite often I am asked, "What is the key to discovering ones purpose?"

I have heard many approaches to the answer this question like asking oneself, "What kind of work, or involved activity would I do for free?" Or if you pay attention to the things that you are able to do that may be challenging to others yet comes with relative ease to you. There is a fundamental difference between discovering one's passion and gifts versus being aligned with true purpose.

The everyday struggle that presents itself is like unto an algebraic expression that needs to be solved. It's designed to unlock yet another small component towards a purpose. This struggle comes in many forms. For example, changing your belief system when found to be both incorrect and inadequate can prove to be true struggle. Our belief leads to emotional responses which in turn lead to action or inaction.

Another way struggle manifests itself is in what has been termed paralysis of analysis, which leads to over thinking and failure to make a decision. Mental struggle may be one of the greatest challenges to overcome. The Inability to halt past experiences, stopping them from becoming current beliefs and ideals of who we are in the present produces suffering.

If you want to study a success story in order to extract the key components, you must take the said subjects struggles prior to the end conclusion under perusal. The reality of struggle can embody hundreds of different word forms ranging from conflict, oppression, and drive to revolution and pain. If we could draw a dividing line to illustrate the point where success and failure happens I would argue that how we view and engage our struggle would be that line. To turn away from our struggle in attempts to avoid the pain and discomfort we associate with it, we in turn miss our opportunity for growth and development.

The Second Law of Thermodynamics explains that entropy, or disorder, increases with time. I know what you're thinking. "What on earth does that have to do with struggle?" Okay allow me to make it plain. Let's say you drop and break a glass of milk on a hard surface, causing it to shatter into thousands of pieces, then you try to gather the substance and all the original pieces and assemble it back together in its original form. It merely takes seconds for the glass of milk to fall and break. However, it could easily take infinity to reverse the action. According to this law, time appears to favor disorder.

This can also be illustrated with the example of the time it takes to clean your home. We often take the time to meticulously put everything in a particular order. Then here comes the family and in a fraction of the time things are back in a disorderly state. The reality is there are more disorderly states in the universe than there are orderly. This can help us understand why the struggle tends to increase with the right things.

Eating in an unhealthy way is not a struggle. It can even be more convenient and often less expensive. Watching TV is the easier path versus reading a quality book or learning a new language. Talking about positive ideals requires a refinement of ones thinking process, and leads to a progressive result. The contrary to this progressive method would be, engaging in negative talk or gossip leading to bad energy and destructive inactivity.

Throughout history, people have found themselves in some of the most abject conditions in which the struggle threatened to compromise their precious sanity. In these extreme conditions, which may have included everything from human bondage to mind numbing torture, many have resulted in different forms of stoicism, meaning the endurance of pain or hardship without a display of feelings and without complaint.

Sometimes we find ourselves working with jobs we find both toxic and dead ends. So what is it that would make someone stay in such a compromising position? Fear of the perceived struggle that making the change would bring. Struggle is the activating pressure that stirs the soul at its very essence and pushes us toward our purpose. It has the effect of making you feel as though you've lost, or that all chips are down. Struggle leaves in its active trail more questions than answers. Questions like "Why me?" "What have I done to deserve this?" "Wow, what next?" and many more. The bottom line is struggle is a complex interwoven part of our existence, but I believe God's purpose for this spiritual opponent is to bring the best out of us. If we rise to the challenge and not acquiesce, it can serve as our guide towards discovering our true purpose.

One of the most powerful tools at our disposal to manage our struggle is gratitude. It is pivotal for success in our walk to be mindful of the many things we have to be grateful for, and take time to acknowledge them. A deep sense of gratitude can put any struggle in its right perspective and secure the boldest inner security of knowing, "This too shall pass".

There is truth in the metaphor, "knowing is half the battle." Knowledge is power. It is a tool designed to fight one of life's costliest opponent - ignorance.

"To whom much is given, much is required."

A bird is not born with the ability to reason. Mama bird does not have the need to teach her new little chicks how to find worms or what to eat for that matter. There are no classes on how to build a nest. They don't just operate from a generic template. If they did all birds would build nest the same way, but they don't. Science has shown they actually learn from their own experience. God gave them an internal blueprint in the form of instinct as with all animals in the kingdom.

This seems like a very efficient deal. An ant cannot go outside of its nature. It simply has to do what it's born to do...period. If you want to test this theory, find some ants and observe them. Watch to see if any ant ever becomes idle or off task.

Now on the other hand, when the beneficent God created man He used an altogether different design. Fashioning man after Himself with the ability to reason, think, imagine, and then bring into existence what is imagined. With these incredible gifts, a man becomes both top caretaker and predator of the animal kingdom. He is the only creature that can go against the very nature he was created in. Unlike the bird, man can decide to eat things he is not even designed to eat. There are parts of the human make up that the individual does not have autonomy over. When there is a set of connected things or parts forming a complex whole, we call it a system.

Due to the extreme, and I do emphasize the extreme, complexity of the electromagnetic vehicle we term as body. God has very brilliantly designated certain functions to be organized into a power system that is governed by an inner intelligence. This system operates without direct awareness of the mind source. The Medulla oblongata for example controls our heartbeat, breathing, blood pressure, and digestion without input from the conscience mind.

This is where the man is given the pathway to greatness. With most of the physical body organized into complex systems and maintained by the inner intelligence, this in turn frees the mental and spiritual mechanisms to manifest man's higher purpose.

When things operate according to a righteous system, balance and harmony is the result. There are similarities between what scientists have named the Milky Way and man's physical composition. There are nine planets in our solar system (some say eight). The sun is the power that draws all the planets into orbit. The magnetic power lies within the light that is emitted from the sun which carries essential life giving properties to the earth. Without this invisible electromagnetic radiation given off by the sun, there could be no life on our planet.

It is truly amazing that all nine planets are engaged in two motions. One is rotating on their own axis at terrific speeds, while the other is simultaneously evolving around the sun. Nine planets all of enormous size is suspended in mid-space without being held up by pillars, only magnetic attraction of the sun. The motions of the heavenly bodies making evolutions around the sun actually create what we know as time. Our earthly body like its heavenly counterpart benefits from nine dynamic planetary systems (organs) revolving around the sun (brain) circulatory, digestive, endocrine, immune system, lymphatic, skeletal nervous, reproductive, and respiratory systems. These systems include all the major and minor organs organized in such a way as to maximize the awesome functioning of the whole organism. The brain is the command system for the entire body similar to the role of the sun in the cosmic context "as above, so below."

As magnificent as this electromagnetic vehicle is, to work at its optimal levels, it must be aligned with the electro-magnetic currents or thoughts. To be ignorant as to how the body works, or even worse, uninterested can prove to be a grave error. Even though there is an inner intelligence designed to perfection, it must be aided with conscience thought to reach a harmonious balance.

A great example of this is iron, which is a part of all cells and has various functions. Iron, which is part of the protein hemoglobin carries oxygen from our lungs throughout our bodies. Having too little hemoglobin is called anemia. Not only does the iron help deliver oxygen to virtually every cell, it also binds with the carbon dioxide which it then transports back to the lung where it is exhaled. So as we can see clearly our inner intelligence knows what to do internally. But due to the fact that our bodies do not produce iron on its own it becomes vital that our conscious mind seeks whole foods rich in iron. We must align our inner intelligence with our conscious thought. This requires that we submit to the idea of eating to live and eating on purpose. We must take the time to educate ourselves on foods and what essential nutrients are held within its essence. The further anything in the plant or animal kingdom gets from its original essence, the less capable it becomes to carry out its unique function. We all should be mindful of this reality if we are interested in reaching optimum holistic health.

One of the reasons I enjoy drawing parallels to the cosmos is because of the beautiful harmony in which it functions. Just imagine that right now we are on this giant rock suspended in space without any pillars holding it up only the sun's magnetism or force. At the same time, we are spinning at the terrific speed of 1037 and 1/3 miles per hour, yet here on the surface without special tools, we can't determine that the earth is even moving at all. In order for this to occur, there must be all but perfect harmony in this solar system.

CHAPTER 7

FITNESS

My son once asked me, "Dad, if you could have any super power what would you choose?" My response was, "wow that's tough since I already possess so many." As you could imagine he looked puzzled.

Well let's explore this. The focusing muscles of the eyes move around 100,000 times a day. The eyes also receive approximately 90 percent of all our information. Who needs X-ray vision with these amazing eyes? Pound for pound bone is stronger than steel, much less dense, but definitely stronger material. When we take time and study our bodies, it is truly amazing.

God has designed our physical compositions so masterfully. We may never discover all the science involved in the makeup. What I wanted my son to understand is once you really take the human body under study, you will find it contains many of the super powers we imagine.

I am a strong advocate of fitness. Why would we not want to reach optimum health through eating right and exercise? Often I observe people approach fitness from a goal oriented incentive. They are motivated to action by a specific set of goals when those goals are:

a) obtained to desired results,

or

b) don't seem to be getting anywhere they simply quit.

Fitness is so much more than a quick scheme to drop some pounds or pack on some powerful looking muscle. The goals are indeed worthy of motivation, but limited in the scope of what total fitness can offer.

There are seven key components of holistic health, fitness, and mental well-being. They are:

1. Cardiovascular/ aerobic conditioning
2. Stretching muscles, ligaments, and tendons
3. Strength training and muscular development
4. Core stability
5. Nutrition and supplementation
6. Mental rest and relaxation
7. Sleep

I will briefly touch on these components. The goal of aerobic activities is to raise your heart rate to your target heart rate. Your maximum heart rate will depend on your age. You can find this number easy. There are many benefits of aerobic exercise, of course combined with a balanced diet, it helps you lose weight and keep it off. It strengthens your heart so it doesn't need to beat as fast, lowers blood pressure and reduces bad cholesterol, lessening the risk of heart attack. The list of benefits goes on and on.

Strength training improves your health in several ways. More muscle mass increases your metabolism, helping you burn more calories, and clears the path for weight control. Weight training also helps bone health. Bone density is at its height at about age thirty. A person loses about a half of a pound of muscle every year after the age of 20, if not actively training. Stretching should be done when muscles, tendons, and ligaments are properly warmed up. Let me be clear here. I am not a professional trainer. Much of what I have learned has been a result of research, trial, and error. My personal favorite form of exercise is calisthenics. Another way of describing calisthenics is bodyweight exercises. I have found calisthenics to be much healthier for the overall body. This form of exercise relies heavily on the core for the explosive poser to complete the exercise.

It's amazing to watch the way these bodyweight exercises reshape the physical composition. There are many goals that can be obtained through working out with weight loss ranking very high on the list or just achieving optimum health in general.

There is another beautiful fruit of labor called the aesthetics of a calisthenics body. One becomes ripped with muscular build, erect posture, balanced development, and best of all no superfluous body fat. A traditional gym is not a necessity. I often work out at a park close to my house. This allows me to get a complete body and mind workout and simultaneously get plenty of sunshine!

The reality is this world we find ourselves in today has become totally laced with a barrage of new technology, constantly vying for our precious attention. It is not unusual to see an entire party out to dinner and everyone is on their smart phones zoned out. Then we have by far become a nation of consumers and the demand has never been higher. True happiness in this kind of reality becomes ever so elusive being replaced instead by tremendous stress, and a new improved version of the rat race. The stress that is the result of this high touch reality can have devastating effects on our health. Surfing the internet does not qualify as cardio! It's imperative that we find time to put aside smart phones tablets, and yes THE GRIND, substituting that time with a hearty workout instead.

The word stress has its origin in both Latin "strictus" (meaning drawn tight), and old French "estresse" (meaning narrowness, oppression). I think the topic of stress deserves our attention. When we are children, we begin experiencing events of how we see ourselves or the world around us can determine how events affects us.

A good example of this is when a child does not receive enough love and affection at home. Not only will they be off balance in how they deal with those outside their home, but they will wear the love bankruptcy on their continence. This rejection of love and affection registers as a form of stress or low self-esteem. This often causes the said individual to gravitate to the negative or lean toward the pessimistic understanding. This powerful noun stresses if left unchecked will take on a life of its own. In an attempt to avoid perceived pain and discomfort, patterns are formed and behavior is modified. In other words, your body records both the negative and positive events that take place in your life. The key lies in the ability to first identify the root causes and how they have impacted you. (I would recommend counseling in some cases.) At some point, we must replace the negative with positive affirmations. Any doctor worth their salt will tell you appropriate exercise can aid in the process of reducing this vicious stress, and they are point on!

I often hear my friends complain that their energy is low. They ask me "What do you do to maintain such high levels of energy?" My response is oxygen and endorphins. This response usually creates a sideways glance as if to say ok back to reality please. Where some of the confusion comes into play is with the seemingly contradicting actions of expending energy in exercise in exchange, receiving energy. In other words, if I'm tired to start with, wouldn't expending my precious limited reserve of energy make me even more tired? That hypothesis seems somewhat logical, albeit this phenomenal body has a different response.

When engaged in exercise, the heart rate is increased and blood is pumped more rapidly throughout the body. Oxygen is then carried to the cells which are converted into energy. Now the next level requires anaerobic exertion. This is a workout so intense the body begins to operate at such a high level that the muscles scream for oxygen. This is often referred to as "runners high". Endorphins are released only at this anaerobic exertion level. This brain chemical is a natural pain and stress fighter. It is this awesome stimulant that leaves one feeling happy and rejuvenated after an intense workout. I guess the old adage "no pain, no gain" has layers of meaning. The bottom line is regardless of your financial position or the different challenges life presents, taking time out to get some good clean exercise is doable.

I often joke with my wife and say you can have the best diet on the planet, but you still have to move something! There simply is no substitute for getting that heart rate up, allowing those lungs to expand and contract, and the skin to release the harmful toxins through sweating. Oh what a feeling!

MOST HIGH GOD

Oh my my my this beautiful body I am in;
Layers of complexity and mystery to no end.
Super heroes with magical powers created
From the imagination from within!
Sometimes I close the windows to my soul
Becoming one with the consciousness
Expressed as I become the goal.

Words can't describe the elation I experience
To feel God's presence with me.
Please, allow me to be a vehicle that you use
To exercise your will through.

What I consider to be freedom
is to be mighty in your kingdom.
King of kings; Lord of lords!
Is this reality not plain enough for
the worldly man to absorb?

Cannot they see the power source of flesh and blood?
How futile it is to worship that which will return to mud.
Well not I,-My praises belong to the Most High!

- Rashon D. Fuller

SECTION 3
GOC

CHAPTER

1

GENESIS OF CHANGE AKA GOC

Before there was GOC, there was Patti.
I'll allow her to share her own story...

I am 3 lbs. away from reaching my goal of losing one hundred pounds in one year!!! *Yes 100 lbs.*

It was the very end of December 2013, as I stared at the phone, awaiting the returned text.

Tina had promised to send some me some juice recipes. On Instagram, I'd seen some of her post which included vibrant photos of the most amazing food and colorful juices and smoothies. Juicing seemed to be the current rave, so I decided I would give it a chance. Who knows...maybe it could jump start my weight loss.

While waiting for the text, I started to think about how I have always looked up to Tina. She'd been my hairstylist from middle school to my senior year of high school, but then she moved away.

She was like a big sister to me and my sisters, Esther and Shanetta. We could tell her anything, and we did! She always listened with genuine care and gave us sound advice about how to navigate this beautiful struggle called LIFE. She inspired us to see our beauty and to understand our self-worth. She also taught us to recognize fire, so we wouldn't get burnt. Simply put, we were schooled on the games boys play.

I was mid thought when the text message finally pinged! Once I opened it,

A BOLD PERSPECTIVE

I realized I had received more than a message containing juice recipes. Instead, I had received a never-ending scribe. She sent me a text report detailing foods that I should include in my daily regimen and foods that I should eliminate. The entire message emphasized living a HEALTHY lifestyle.

At first glance, I knew I wasn't going to do 70% of what was listed. I honestly wanted to do things my way. Yet, deep down inside, I knew I had to do something different in order to yield different results.

I had to make changes, and I had to do it quickly. I was quickly approaching my heaviest weight.

I was frustrated, stressed, and overall unhappy! I would diet for 3 or 4 months with success, but would gain all the weight back... The cycle was recurring and depression became a constant companion. I had very little desire to do anything outside of work.

While sitting in the house, I would bore quickly, so I ate. Food seemed to be the only thing that satisfied my feelings of depression and boredom. At some point, my inner consciousness realized that this was no way to live and I wanted out of this lifelong cycle. I was days away from the New Year, and I made a resolution that 2014 was the year I would get my health back

IT WAS MY TIME FOR CHANGE, so I took action!

Every morning I look in the mirror and greet myself with "Sawubona, Skihona." The South African Zoulous Tribe greets each other with "Sawubona, Sikhona" which translates into English as "*I SEE YOU, I AM HERE.*" In other words, when you acknowledge your presence then you exist.

Despite feeling skinny, fat, unattractive or broken, I acknowledge MY PRESENCE as I am.

I am the mirror image of the Creator and I EXIST!

After the first two weeks of following the scribe, I lost over 10 lbs. My migraines decreased significantly, from 1 every day to 2 a week. Within 6 weeks, I had lost over 20 lbs. and I felt great! I was so proud of me and there was light at the end of the tunnel. Within the first quarter of my lifestyle change, I had an epiphany....what if I worked out, too? I could possibly reach my goal quicker. So I got a trainer! For four days a week I was in "beast mode" and trained for an hour.

Every day was a struggle, especially going to the gym, but I stayed focused and press forward. Each day I make a concerted effort not to engage in "stress-eating". Instead, I manage my emotions and stress levels, and I made better lifestyle decisions when I confront the two. I unraveled a lifetime of bad habits… but every step of the way has been worth it!

ELEVEN MONTHS AND TWO WEEKS LATER…

It only took me 2 weeks to come out of pre-hypertension after changing my *lifestyle*.

My doctor visits no longer include diabetes checks. My blood pressure has been consistently normal, and I have a better quality of life! The journey has proven to be so much more than just weight loss, it has been mental, emotional, physical, and even spiritual. I've made healthy choices and I am saving my life. The initial stages of change are never easy, but I AM WORTH IT!

One day I woke up and decided I would be beautiful. I would live a beautiful life. I wasn't going to wait on Skinny. I was going to have fun, go out, travel, live, move and be kind. I'm going to smile and look people in the eye when I speak to them. One day I decided to let my soul open up for the world to see and be ok with that vulnerability. My life started in that moment!

If skinny came, it would be at her own pace. She is no longer going to dictate my future, be the answer to my prayers or my only road to happiness. I am no longer willing to accept that formulation.

Recently, I was asked, "What is my total weight goal?"

Well…

I don't have a final weight goal because it's daunting…. but my fitness goals are to compete a 5K OBSTACLE COURSE, to RIDE 2 miles on my bike… I also want to be 70% raw 90% of the time… and those goals will get me in my right size body whatever that is… LOL

As of now I am now 3 lbs. away from my goal of losing 100 lbs. in one year and there is still 2 weeks left until the year ends.

Tina, of the gifts that you have given me, the greatest is eating God's way!

You never asked me to count calories, carbohydrates, or add up points. You simply taught me nutritional balance. Now I have increased confidence, energy, beautiful skin and NO MORE MIGRAINES!

There is no way I can ever repay you, but do know, I love you and I hope to one day inspire and impact one person's life the way you have my mine.

I am *Patricia Dorsey* and I AM HERE!

CHAPTER

2

BACK TO THE BASICS

*DISCLAIMER

Before starting any major dietary changes, it is important to consult with your doctor first. This is especially important if you have any medical conditions.

We are not Doctors, Nutritionist or Chefs. We are just a couple who decided to take charge of our health through nutrition wellness.

However, we have feedback from a doctor...

This GOC journey was an excellent experience! As a former fitness competitor through hard work and discipline I had achieved my goals. But looking back my meals plans were unbalanced and very restrictive. Often times these plans included high daily protein requirements of 4-5 portions of lean meat with few varieties of vegetables and little to no fruit.

This way of eating was reinforced by the physique I achieved and rewarded by my trophies. I competed in 5 shows and I have won 5 trophies! *Of all my victories my most prized moment was winning 1st place in the NPC* (National Physique Committee) in California in front of my family and friends!

But at some point, I forgot how-to eat without labeling food as "good" or "bad" or as a "cheat".

After two years of not competing I was still unable to reprogram my relationship with food.

When asked to review GOC from a physician/health perspective I asked Tina if

A BOLD PERSPECTIVE

I could try the program, so that I may give an honest opinion.

Within the first week which was the *cleanse and vegan* part of the journey, my refrigerator and *my life was changed for the better.* There was so much color and variety with so many options of food combinations! As I chopped vegetables, my kitchen counter was vibrant and full of life!

The fitness nut in me still needed to know my macronutrient intake and found by plugging the recipes into my preferred program myfitnesspal.com, that I was also getting a good balance!

On my chart Health + Balance = Win/Win!

During my 21 days of GOC I continued a strenuous training programs with my personal trainer. I felt strong, full of energy and my digestive system enjoyed the journey too!

Since finishing GOC I find myself reading more about plant-based proteins. I am confident that I am on my way to once again achieving my health and fitness goals, but in a Healthy, Balanced and Sustainable way!

Thank you for the opportunity to walk this path of GOC!!!

P.s My personal goal for this journey was to reset my relationship with food developing a healthy and mental attitude toward all that nature has to offer. I achieved that and so much more!

-Ayana Baker, MD

People are constantly puzzled by our nutritional lifestyle, *as if the way that we eat is new…*

The reality is the Western diet of burgers, fries, pizza, soda, daily animal products, sugar, processed and "fried everything" that most people consume daily is a fairly new way of life. Our ancestors certainly didn't eat the way many of us do today. Their diets were devoid of pesticides, additives, genetically modified foods, and artificial flavors, etc… This new way of eating was adopted by our modern culture and is responsible for distorting and destroying our bodies. Research shows that life expectancy has increased, but we are sick to death and surviving on meds. If you ask us, (The Fuller's) *that's no way to live.*

In order to reverse and prevent the illnesses that our nation is experiencing, we must **GO BACK TO THE BASICS**!

What are the basics, you may ask…**NUTRIENTS**!

REMEMBER…

One of the first things that God told mankind is what to eat and what not to eat. *Eating the wrong thing has been getting us in trouble since the beginning of time. Remember…?* The first curse of mankind was released due to eating the wrong thing.

-Tomorrow Dawn

DEAR JOURNAL   March 20, 2012 a.m.

Today I am meeting with Mrs. Olivette, an 83-year-old woman who is like a grandmother to my husband. For close to a year now, he's been urging me to just have a sit down with her. He declares that one day after taking very ill and barely being able to stand he called her and she immediately sent him a taxi that delivered him to her home. Upon arriving, she gave him her bed for 3 days and nursed him to a place that he said he had never been. He said the degree of energy and clearness of mind, he experienced was unimaginable! What he calls green and white smoothies were the only foods that she gave him during his 3 day stay.

RA says her community comes to her aid for many health issues. He has spoken of one individual who came to her home in the advanced stages of cancer, after being under her care for some time once returning to the doctor they could not find a trace of cancer. So off I go.

DEAR JOURNAL March 20, 2012 p.m.

WHY HAVE I WAITED SO LONG TO MEET THIS SWEET and FEISTY WOMAN! This woman's knowledge of the body and how it responds to food is amazing! Her humor, her wit, and wisdom are just outstanding. I think I've found my mentor!

During my meeting with Mrs. Olivevette, she blessed me with jewels to add to the path that we had begun a year ago.

1. Amino Acids are equivalent to protein! Amino Acids are the building blocks for protein, which means the body can receive proper and sufficient protein from plant-based food groups such as veggies, grains, lentils, beans, nuts, and fruits.
2. The ONLY two reasons why people should eat
   1. Energy 2. To Repair tissue and cells.

Most people feed their bodies with foods that are of empty nutrients (I was very guilty) and foods that the body cannot benefit from. "-But it tastes good though becomes our reasoning."

The occupants of our country are paying dearly with their health due to deficiency of proper nutrition. We are full in the belly, but yet our bodies are starved of nutrients. Just look at how many people have high blood pressure, high cholesterol, cancer and weight issues, just to name a few.

3. Foods with Sulfur purifies the body. Sulfur rich foods are cabbage, cauliflower, onions, broccoli, garlic, brazil nuts and walnuts.
4. Pineapple and Papaya both have natural enzymes to assist the body with digestion and should be eaten, especially after eating the meat, dairy, and whites (flour, bread, rice and so forth)
5. Avocado and Grapes are excellent sources of Iron.
6. Watercress, Chick Peas, and Sunflower Sprouts are excellent hormone balancers.
7. Natural Antibiotics foods are Asparagus, Cabbage, Garlic, Parsley, and Watercress.

WOW! After filling my journal with all of this PRO-LIFE information that she rolled of her tongue, I asked Mrs. Olivette if she could Only eat 12 food items what would they be?

Her response was, *"I'll go for the most powerful ones!"*

Her list went as follows: avocado, grapes, kiwi, blue and blackberries, cherries, broccoli, sunflower seeds, sesame seeds, pumpkin seeds, almonds, cumin, and apples. Yeah, she went over 12 items, but was okay with that. I brought my journal, I came to learn!

Before leaving Mrs. Olivette's home, she suggested I should get going on a 28 day fast, utilizing only a purifying juice (with main ingredients cauliflower and lime) and salads. She also urged me to load my salads with leafy greens, fruit, seeds, nuts, and asparagus. For salad dressing, her recommendation was fresh lime juice.

So I looked at her kind of sideways, because this seemed extreme.

Then I asked, "You eat asparagus raw?"

"R A W" She replied,

"What do you mean raw? Don't you know when the good Lord shined his sunshine on it, he cooked it to Perfection. You take it home and over cook it!"

A BOLD PERSPECTIVE

I laughed and asked well, "Can I add a little sea salt to the dressing?"

To which she replied, "Baby, you can take that sea salt and either put it in your bath to soak or throw it back in the ocean!"

Before I left she dropped one last jewel.

We are electromagnetic beings, which makes us powerful energy. Our bodies don't need to know the name of the problem to fix itself, as it is self-sufficient and operates on its own intelligence. Our bodies just need the proper energy [foods] to correct the problem.

Needless to say, I was blown away.

Thank You Mrs. Olivette, for *teaching* Nutritional Wellness!

NUTRIENTS: *the nutritious components in foods that an organism utilizes to survive and grow.*

Nutrients are used to repair tissues, regulate body processes, and are converted to and used for energy. Plants by way of fruits and vegetables intake nutrients directly from the sun and soil, and is absorbed through roots and leaves. As we eat these plants based foods we consume nutrients.

The 6 main groups of *nutrients* are *vitamins, minerals, carbs, fats, protein* and *water*.

Below are a list of phytonutrients (*plant based foods*).

Healthy sources of **Vitamins** *and* **Minerals** *are found in:*

- Fruits
- Vegetables

Healthy **Carbs** *are found in:*

- Fruit
- Vegetables

- Legumes
- Nuts and Seeds
- Unrefined Whole Grains: brown rice, quinoa, barley, bulgur, wild rice, oats, buckwheat, whole wheat, and whole rye.

*Healthy **Fats** are found in:*

- Avocado
- Olive oil
- Sunflower oil
- Sesame oil
- Avocados
- Olives
- Nuts
- Nut butter
- Seeds: sesame, pumpkin, hemp, flax, sunflower

*Healthy **Proteins** are found in:*
Nut/Seed (grams of protein per 1/4 Cup or 4 tbs)
Chia Seed   12
Hemp Seed 10
Flax Seed 8
Sunflower Seed 8
Sala 7.4
Almond 7
Pumpkin Seed 7
Sesame Seed 7
Pistachio 6
Walnut 5
Brazil Nut 5

Hazelnut 5
Pine Nut 4
Cashew 4
Beans ((grams of protein per 1 Cup cooked))
Lentil 18
Adzuki 17
Cannellini (white beans) 17
Cranberry bean 17
Navy Bean 16
Split Peas 16
Anasazi 15
Black Bean 15
Garbanzos (chick peas) 15
Kidney Bean 15
Great Northern Beans 15
Lima Beans 15
Pink Beans 15
Black-eyed Peas 14
Mung Beans 14
Pinto Beans 14
Green Peas 9
Grain (grams of protein per 1 Cup cooked)
Triticale 25
Millet 8.4
Amaranth 7
Oat, bran 7
Wild Rice 7
Rye Berries 7
Whole Wheat Couscous 6
Bulgur Wheat 6

Buckwheat 6
Tiff 6
Oat Grouts 6
Barley 5
Quinoa 5
Brown Rice 5
Spelt 5
Vegetables (grams of protein per quantity size)
Corn (1 large cob) 5
Potato (with skin) 5
Mushroom, Oyster (1 cup) 5
Collard Greens (1 cup) 4
Peas (1/2 cup) 4
Artichoke (medium) 4
Broccoli (1 cup) 4
Brussels sprouts (1 cup) 4
Mushroom, Shitake (1 cup) 3.5
Fennel (1 medium bulb) 3
Swiss chard (1 cup) 3
Kale (1 cup) 2.5
Asparagus (5 spears) 2
String Beans (1 cup) 2
Beets (1 cup) 2
Sweet Potato (1 cup) 3
Cabbage (1 cup) 2
Carrot (1 cup) 2
Cauliflower (1 cup) 2
Rutabaga 2
Squash 2
Celery (1 cup) 1

Spinach (1 cup) 1
Bell Peppers (1 cup) 1
Cucumber (1 cup 1
Eggplant (1 cup) 1
Leeks (1 cup) 1
Lettuce (1 cup) 1
Okra (1/2 cup) 1
Onion (1/2 cup) 1

And let's not forget *WATER*

Water is our Life Line! The human body is composed of 75% water. Without water our bodies are equivalent to a dehydrated plant. When a plant is in need of water and doesn't receive it, dehydration set in. The plant's leaves lose its firmness. The soft leaves are the plant losing its life aka ENERGY. If the plant continues to receive no water eventually it will expire. But, if the plant receives water and sunlight that same plant can be restored. Our bodies operate in a similar manner.

CHAPTER 3

THE JOURNEY

GOC

What exactly is GOC? It is short for GENESIS OF CHANGE. What is the purpose of this genesis? We need a new beginning because it is now more important than ever for us to take control of our health. ***Our lives matter!***

How it Began...

We, Tina and Rashon Fuller, are advocates who believe that animal products should ONLY be eaten in moderation, or not at all. WHY? Well, animal-based foods are one of the main culprits behind our nation's top three causes of death.

We believe that the daily consumption of food should consist of eighty percent plant-based nutrients aka phytonutrients. Plant based nutrients are power-packed with vitamins and minerals which positively impact our bodies.

After having many conversations with dozens of people, we found that the hardest part, of achieving a healthy lifestyle, seemed to be getting started. Our solution to an easier start is to start with a team and adopt an outlined [nutrition] plan! In a team, you have accountability partners. A team effort is always more exciting than the efforts of an individual. And as part of a team, we push and pull one another through to the finish line.

One evening, while Rashon and I were at the dining room table finishing up dinner, he initiated a conversation that went a little something like this...

"I know people who are ready to transition to a healthier lifestyle. They are standing at the scratch line, but with so much conflicting information they don't know where to start."

He went on to say, "What if we organized a group and created a health challenge? We could provide parameters for healthy food choices and maybe even a workout regimen. This could be really effective! It may just be what people need. We could provide the tools to help jumpstart a healthy transition into nutritional wellness."

Rashon added, "Tina, think about it... how often have we seen people lose weight. They look great and say they feel great, but within a year or so, they've regained all their weight and more? The problem is not their lack of dedication. The problem is that very few people can actually live on a diet."

He was right. The moment a diet is altered from its rigorous plan, the mind begins to crave everything that was previously forbidden. This can lead to the onset of a vicious cycle of binge eating.

After breaking a diet, the original lifestyle is back with a vengeance, in no time. Down the drain goes all the sacrifice. And not to mention, weight fluctuation and obesity are not the only problems... they're not even the biggest problems.

With the Standard American Diet (SAD) being at the root of so much sickness, disease, and even death, Rashon suggested that we create a 21-day challenge!

We wanted to make a difference that could help teach people to live a sustainable lifestyle. As you may have guessed, Rashon suggested that we call the challenge "Genesis of Change!" Everything he said was like music to my soul. And just like that, I was sold!

With this in mind, Rashon and I began journeying through vegan, vegetarian, pescetarian, and 80/20 lifestyles. Straight away, I took the idea and started journaling a plan. Within a few days, I had a full outline and it was totally centered around nutritional balance. I presented it to Rashon, and he approved!

So, here you have it... GOC!!!

Getting Organized

After creating the total layout, I knew that we needed a team. So, I pondered the best way to organize a team and social media seemed to be the most effective route. On my Instagram and Facebook pages, I made the following post:

To complete our Genesis of Change team, we would like a total of 12 people. What is Genesis of Change? It is *charity, accountability,* and a *21-day food journey challenge.* The 21 days will come with daily recipes and a weekly grocery-shopping list. You must be local (Atlanta) and you must be ready for change.

We ended up with 16 people!!!

Soon, I followed up with an email to everyone that read:

The rest is history!

The Journey: Nutritional Guidelines

This food journey is broken down into multiple "foodie" lifestyle categories.

- ☐ 1 day of cleansing (fruits and veggies)
- ☐ 5 days of a vegan lifestyle (100% plant based: fruits, veggies, whole grains, beans, nuts, and seeds)
- ☐ 5 days of a vegetarian lifestyle (fruits, veggies, whole grains, beans, nuts, seeds, bread [optional: cheese and eggs])
- ☐ 5 days of a pescetarian lifestyle (fruits, veggies, whole grains, nuts, seeds, beans, bread [optional: seafood])
- ☐ 5 days of an 80/20 lifestyle (80% fruits, veggies, whole grains, nuts, seeds, beans, bread [optional: 20% seafood, poultry, eggs, and cheese])

Note: *If you are totally vegan, no worries! Simple alterations will keep you in the game.*

If you are new to all of this, don't stress. Our recipes are simple, flavorful, and satisfying!

During the 80/20 period, two of the five days include the option of eating animal-based products.

Having an outlined plan is vital, because it removes the guesswork from the daunting task of determining what to eat each day.

Our 21-day journey includes a weekly grocery-shopping list for:

- ☐ Breakfast and lunch options, with recipes
- ☐ Smoothie and snack options, with recipes
- ☐ 21 Dinner recipes, with appetizing photos (photos on the website)

An added bonus to the journey is the use of group chat. Group chat should be established for your team, we recommend using Group Me. This can be your team's direct line of communication with one another. You can share pics of your food, share your workout regimens, words of encouragement, health tips, and even questions.

Additionally, we encourage you to pick a few days and workout as a group. It could be a 30-minute walk in the park, yoga, kickball, Zumba, basketball, bike riding, or a light jog. If gathering a group becomes mission impossible, still move forward even if it's an individual effort.

PROOF IS IN THE NUMBERS

Just a little added insight…

The top three causes of death in America are:

1. Heart Disease 596,577
2. Cancer 576,691
3. Chronic Lower Respiratory Disease 142,943

Death totals from one year.

Chronic diseases and conditions—such as heart disease, stroke, cancer, diabetes, obesity, and arthritis—are among the most common, costly, and preventable of all health problems.

- As of 2012, about half of all adults—117 million people—have one or more chronic health conditions. One of the four adults has two or more chronic health conditions.

- The number of deaths in the US in 2010 was 2,515,458. Together heart disease and cancer accounted for 48% of all deaths.

- Obesity is a serious health concern. During 2009–2010, more than one-third of adults or about 78 million people, were obese (defined as body mass index [BMI] ≥30 kg/m2). Nearly one of five youths aged 2–19 years was obese (BMI ≥95th percentile).

- Arthritis is the most common cause of disability. Of the 53 million adults with a doctor diagnosis of arthritis, more than 22 million say arthritis causes them to have trouble with their usual activities.

- Diabetes is the leading cause of kidney failure, lower limb amputations other than those caused by injury, and new cases of blindness among adults.

- About half of US adults (47%) have at least one of the following major risk factors for heart disease or stroke: uncontrolled high blood pressure, uncontrolled high LDL cholesterol, or are current smokers. Ninety percent of Americans consume too much sodium, increasing their risk of high blood pressure.

All three of these conditions share a common denominator, they are preventable.

Here are a few additional benefits and reasons to eat well:

- INCREASED ENERGY
- NATURAL BODY WEIGHT
- STRIKING NATURAL GLOW
- CLARITY OF MIND
- NATURAL BALANCE
- DECREASED JUNK FOOD CRAVINGS
- TOTAL IMMUNE SYSTEM BOOST
- A NEW LEVEL OF CONSCIOUSNESS
- INCREASED ALKALINITY BALANCE
- BETTER BOWEL MOVEMENTS *which prevent the body from storing waste that contributes to sickness.*

And just in case those reasons aren't enough, *a healthy nutritional lifestyle can help prolong your youthful appearance and longevity!*

The Challenge: Rules of Engagement

Ultimately, we are collectively one group GOC and we have one goal, and that's nutritional wellness. However, we recommend forming a GOC group of your own. Your group may vary from as small as 4 people, with you included. Or your group may be as large as 40 people or more. Be sure to have an even number.

Then, this group should be split into two even sub-teams, Team A and Team B. Feel free to personalize your group with a sub-name. Depending on where and how the group is formed, it may predetermine the group's name.

For example: If your book club, church, job, or whatever your group… decides to do the challenge together. The group members may decide to name the group after that organization. This is what Rashon and I did, we named our group after our business. We were GOC Teams A and B of Zero Gravity.

The day before the challenge begins, your full group should meet in order to:

1. Waist-in (measure the waist of each person)
2. Split into the two smaller sub-teams (Team A and Team B)
3. Provide group chat information to both sub-teams, with instructions. Even though, the group is split in two, we recommend both sub-teams being on the same (one) group chat.
4. MAKE IT BEAUTIFUL! Collect a donation from each team member (to be given to charity). Each group can decide their donation amount. We decided on $20 per person. But, feel free to donate more…

Sub-teams can be chosen by randomly pulling a letter from a box or hat. Once sub-teams have been determined, donations have been collected, and group chat has been established, the challenge can begin.

At the end of the 21-day journey, your group should have a final waist-out.

Every [waist] inch lost equals one point. Half inches count as half a point. Here's an example:

> At the beginning of the challenge, let's say teammate #1 from Team A has a waist that measures at 36". But at the end of the 21-day journey his/her waist measurement is 34" – Team A adds two points to their score! However, if the opposite occurs and your teammate's waist now measures at 37" and at the end she is up from 36", Team A gets one point deducted.

Chose a day to have the waist-out. I would recommend the day after the challenge ends. As schedules get busy, you may allow two days for the waist-out. For those who fail to show for the waist-out, their points won't be able to count, unless your group agrees to allow to a very clear video upload of someone accurately measuring the teammates' waist. The video should show the face and waist measurement of the team member.

In the end, the team with the most points wins! The winning team can select the charity to which funds should be donated. All funds should be donated in the name of Genesis of Change by way of your groups name...

So, that's all folks! Let's begin the journey and enjoy!

Oh yeah, I recommend starting the challenge at the beginning of the week, Sunday.

Frequently Asked Questions

Q | Does it matter how many people are in my group?

A | No, but we recommend selecting an even number.

Q | Can GOC be accomplished on my own?

A | Yes. However, experiencing the journey as a group is better, because it offers support, excitement,

and accountability.

Q | What is the average amount that I should expect to spend on groceries?

A | We highly recommend shopping at farmer's markets for better prices and fresher produce. During the challenge, amongst a group of 16 the average grocery-shopping bill was about $90 per week for 2 adults. Add $20 per adult.

Q | Are we restricted to only eating what's on the menu?

A | No, but we recommend staying within the Nutritional Guidelines developed for the Journey.

Q | Are we allowed to snack?

A | Yes. As a group we created a list of healthy snacks: dried and fresh fruit, granola bars, nuts, homemade popcorn, non-dairy parfaits and leftovers.

Q | Does everyone in the group have to be local?

A | In the beginning, we thought that teammates should be local. However, we learned geography wasn't so important. As long as team members are able to participate via group chat, distance should be fine. We also recommend that each long-distance waist-in and [out] is done via video chat, such as FaceTime, Skype, Hangouts or Emailed video footage.

Q | Can we have coffee?

A | Most coffee drinkers can run down a list of health benefits to building a case for drinking coffee. However, very few know the negative factors. After being asked this question by several GOCer's, we decided to do some research. So, here are the main points that stood out to us:

1. Coffee bean crops are commonly sprayed with pesticides.
2. In the body, coffee can function as a nutrient blocker when consumed in abundance.
3. Coffee can be addictive.
4. Coffee is acidic.

These were a few of the negative results of our research, but we encourage you to do your own. If you find that you simply must have it [coffee], we recommend that you only have one to two cups on the weekend. Let it be your treat to yourself.

Q | Can we have alcohol?

A | No, we recommend abstaining from liquor. However, wine is fine in mild moderation.

Q | Can we eat out?

A | If you must, eat according to the journey. ex: the night of stir-fry, due to a long work day our family ate veggie stir-fry from a local Thai restaurant. We had brown jasmine rice with veggies. We also ate fish tacos out due to another busy work day.

Q | For the day 14 pizza party, can we have real pizza?

A | Yes! We ordered our pizza from a local pizzeria. Rashon and I hosted game night/pizza party at our home. We ordered cheese pizzas plus we made falafels. Our GOC group mates provided the wine and salad.

TESTIMONIALS

At the start of GOC, not once did I think I was about to embark on a journey that would change my life forever.

I enjoyed everything from cooking to reading labels during my farmer's market trips to measuring a cup of coconut milk during meal prep. It was all exciting.

Not to mention my energy levels were off the charts, my cravings for sweets decreased and *weekly I saved an average of $50/week on food*; previously I would overspend on groceries and dining out.

Sheliah

Every married couple should take this journey. GOC has allowed us to become closer and has shown us how to eat healthier as a couple too. Finally, we are now on the same nutritional page!
p.s… *Within two months of GOC, we "naturally" conceived after one year and two months of TTC [Trying to Conceive]!!!*

Duane and Amour

I have learned how to prepare fresh veggies & fruits in a snap. I have learned the 80/20 rule which is the bomb! 80% vegan 20% waste… GOC is a part of the new me!

Melody

In 21 days, *I lost 1-1/2 inches off my waist*!
Thank you for teaching me that it is never too late to make positive changes. From here on out I am forever Genesis of Change.

Mama Val

A BOLD PERSPECTIVE

GOC has taught me the how-to on Eating to Live, not Living to Eat.
I have been a lifelong yo-yo dieter. I have spent unknown amounts of money on destination health spas, hospital sponsored lifestyle change programs, books, etc. In 21 days, I *lost 3 inches* off my waist and 4 pound in weight.
My new DAILY MANTRA...
"My Body is healthy, graceful, and slender"!

Sherida

My personal goals were to have more energy, increased (BM) elimination, lose a few pounds, perhaps gain a smaller waistline and gain some new healthy recipes. *Well, I certainly exceeded all my goals*! To top it all off, I've lost 2.5 inches off my waistline!!

Shandra

I find that most recipes are not in layman's terms and I would have to Google the items in the recipe. Not the case with GOC. *Easy to follow and prepare meals* and easy on my wallet too! Total WIN!

Joy

This eating plan is our new beginning! GOC is not a "diet" *GOC is incredible*! We thoroughly enjoyed this experience and the meals were all tasty!

Marcus and Clarissa

Genesis of Change is the perfect name! Before I started this journey healthy eating seemed boring, bland, and out of my budget. I could not have imagined being satisfied without some type of meat, cheese or bread with every meal.
I embraced this journey head on, with the hopes of just learning a few healthy recipes. *What I received in return was flavorful and exciting meals*, plus 1 ½ inches from my waist!

Artanza

A few mental notes…

DIRTY DOZEN/CLEAN 15

The fruits and vegetables on "The Dirty Dozen" list, when conventionally grown, tested positive for at least 47 to 67 different chemicals. For produce on the "dirty" list, you should definitely Go Organic unless you relish the idea of consuming chemicals.

Dirty Dozen

1. Apples
2. Strawberries
3. Grapes
4. Celery
5. Peaches
6. Spinach
7. Sweet Bell Peppers
8. Nectarines -imported
9. Cucumbers
10. Cherry Tomatoes
11. Snap Peas -imported
12. potatoes

All the produce on "The Clean 15" bore little to no traces of pesticides and is safe to consume in non-organic form.

Clean 15

1. Sweet Potatoes
2. Cauliflower
3. Cantaloupe
4. Grapefruit

5. Eggplant

6. Kiwi

7. Papaya

8. Mangoes

9. Asparagus

10. Onions

11. Sweet Peas -Frozen

12. Cabbage

13. Pineapples

14. Sweet Corn

15. Avocados

GMO's are foods produced from organisms that have had specific changes introduced into their DNA using the methods of genetic engineering. Genetically modified foods have been shown to cause harm to humans, animals, and the environment. GMO's are plants or animals.

Tips: If fruit doesn't have seeds it is not fruit. It is GMO! If the ingredients have the words refined or fortified, it is GMO.

If the produce is certified USDA-organic, it's non-GMO (*or supposed to be.*) To avoid GMO shop with local farmers or start your own organic garden!

Here are the top 10 GMO foods

- Soy
- Corn
- Canola Oil
- Cotton
- Dairy
- Sugar
- Aspartame
- Zucchini
- Yellow Squash
- Papaya grown in Hawaii

The best way to preserve the freshness of berries is to store them in the refrigerator in an airtight container like a mason jar.

CHAPTER 4

WELCOME TO GENESIS OF CHANGE!

Phase one...

"ROLL CALL"... Are You Here? There is no better time to start than now!

We hope that you are as excited as we are, to embark upon this life changing JOURNEY!

Our mission is to become the healthy and knowledgeable human beings that we were created to be.

Items needed to participate in this journey
*COMMITMENT
*DISCIPLINE

Plus...
Week 1
- Blender (We prefer Vitamix. But any quality blender should be fine)
- Wide mouth Mason Jars (We purchase two sizes: one pint and one and a half pint. Jars by Ball)
- Food Processor
- Pots and Pans
- Ice cream scooper (optional)

Week 2
- Shaker Ball for protein shakes.
- A julienne, cheese grater, potato peeler, or a spiral slicer. (We prefer our Spirooli. Purchased from Bed, Bath and Beyond).GENESIS OF CHANGE

Week 3
- Same items from the previous weeks.

DISCLAIMER #2.

IF, I have left anything off the shopping list or the recipe(s) please forgive me and work with me…
I am new to this type of project and it proved to be overwhelming, but I conquered!

Be sure to check for **Meal Preps:** foods that need to be prepped for the next day.
Be sure to visit www.SoLiberating.com *for updated information and images* of the GOC meals.

LETS' GO!

WEEK 1
MENU, Grocery List, and Recipes

Dinner for the week
Big Ole Salad
Lentil Soup
Asian Stir Fry
Asparagus and Mash
Falafel Tacos
Fruit Salad and Smoothie
Stuffed Rolls and Mushrooms

Water is VERY important. It is one of Nature's best cleansers. Be certain to drink no less than 48oz daily.

* All shopping list and recipes are designed for 2 servings/persons. If it is just you in your household purchase half the ingredients and cut the recipes in half. Ex: instead purchasing two green apples purchase one. Instead of using two cups of spinach use one.

WEEK 1 GROCERY LIST

5 gallons Spring Water
1 whole Pineapple
1 Lemon
1 Limes
2 Green Apple
2 Green Pear
2 Red Pears
2 Oranges
Bananas
2 Mangos (frozen is fine if out of season)
Raspberries or strawberries
Dried Cranberries
10 oz. Spring of Red Leaf Lettuce
10 oz. bag of Spinach
1 Bunch of Kale
1 Bunch of Collards (optional for lentil soup)
1 Red Cabbage
1 lb. Green Beans
Sunflower Sprouts (optional for tacos)
1 bag of whole Carrots
2 medium Zucchinis
2 Cucumbers
Celery
1 Avocado
Asparagus

A BOLD PERSPECTIVE

2 Broccoli Crowns
10 Roma Tomatoes
1 large or 2 small Bok Choy
2 Sweet Onions
1 Red Bell Pepper
1 Yellow Bell Pepper
Thyme (fresh)
Cilantro (fresh)
American Basil (fresh)
Rosemary (fresh)
1 whole Garlic
1 Parsley (fresh)
1 small Ginger
2 Packs of Baby Bella Mushrooms
5 medium Red Potatoes
2 Vanilla Coconut Yogurt aka Cultured Coconut Milk
1 Plain Coconut Yogurt
Almond Milk or Almond Coconut Milk
Whole Lentils Brown or Green
Ground Cumin
Cinnamon
Fennel ground or seeds
Sea or Kosher Salt
Black Pepper
Rolls (we prefer crusty roll like French bread. Be sure it has no high fructose corn syrup)
Cheese slices (we prefer Mozzarella or Havarti)
Croutons
Tortilla Shells or Pita Bread
Steel Cut Oats
Old Fashioned Rolled Oats
Chick Peas aka Garbanzo Beans
Rice (we prefer brown Jasmine, wild or black rice)
Teriyaki or Stir Fry Sauce (we prefer Kikkoman sauce, not marinade)
Olive Oil
Maple Syrup
Vanilla extract (optional for oatmeal and granola)

32oz Veggie Broth in a carton (we prefer Swanson)
Wine or Champagne Vinegar
1/4 lb. Raw Almonds
1/4 lb. Raw Cacao aka cocoa nibs (sold cheaper at Farmer's Market...)
Chocolate powder [(like Hershey's) optional for Power RA]
Sesame Seeds (we prefer black)
Veggie Bouillon cubes (we prefer Knorr)
Flour (we prefer all purpose or whole wheat)
(Grab a few extra items for salad ex: cucumbers, tomato, fruit, etc...)

DAY 1 "CLEANSE"
Week 1

1st Meal
GREEN WORKS Smoothie
2 cups of organic Spinach
1 Green Apple (cut and remove seeds)
1/4 cup Fresh Parsley Leaves
1 cup Pineapple
1 1/2" piece of Ginger
1 cup Spring Water
1 cup Ice
Blend.

2nd Meal
Any Fruit 2 whole fruits ex: apple and orange or 2 cups of fresh cut fruit.

3rd Meal
A Big Ole (veggies and/or fruit only) Salad paired anyway you like.
My salad: Spring mix, kale, shredded red Cabbage, Carrots, Cucumbers, Tomatoes, Onions, Pears, Pineapples, and dried Cranberries.

WHY buy salad dressing when you can make your own!

1/4 cup Vinegar (We prefer Champagne, Balsamic, or Wine Vinegar)
1/4 cup of Olive Oil
Juice from 1/2 a orange or a 1/2 a lemon or 1/2 a lime
2 tsp Maple Syrup
1/2 tsp. Garlic Clove diced
1/2 tsp Fresh Thyme leaves
1 tsp Fresh Basil chopped
Dash of Salt
Fresh pepper (We prefer cracked)
Mix and pour

Meal Prep: Tonight overnight (soak) your lentils for tomorrow's soup.
1 cup of Lentils soaked in 2 cups of water.

DAY 2 "VEGAN"
Week 1

1st Meal
SWEET PINK Smoothie
1 Red Pear
12 Raspberries or 6 Strawberries
1 Banana
3 oz. of Vanilla Coconut Yogurt
Juice from 1 Orange
1 cup of water
1 cup of Ice
Blend.

2nd Meal
Mason Jar Salad prepared anyway that you like! I'll repeat yesterday's salad but I'll add berries!
Mason jar Instructions: place desired amount dressing in the bottom of the Mason jar. Layer jar starting with cucumbers, tomatoes then layer the

remaining ingredients. When it's time to eat it, be sure the lid is tightly secured, turn the jar upside down shake, shake, shake and Enjoy!!!

3rd Meal
LENTIL SOUP
32 oz. Veggie broth in a carton
1 cup Lentils
3 cups Collards (may be substituted for kale)
1 medium Carrot
2 Celery Stalks
1 medium Zucchini
1/2 Sweet Onion
4 Roma Tomatoes
Leaves from 3 sprigs of Thyme
A handful Basil leaves
A few Parsley leaves
A few Cilantro leaves
2 Garlic Cloves
2 tsp Olive Oil
1 Tbsp Cumin
Add sea salt and pepper to taste

Instruction:
Chop greens, carrots, celery, zucchini, tomatoes, basil, and parsley.
Dice onions, tomatoes, and garlic
Drain and rinse the lentils.
Combine in a pot broth, lentils, 2 cups of water and 1 bouillon cube. Bring to a boil.
Sauté in a saucepan onions and garlic in olive oil for 5 minutes. Stir in basil, tomatoes and a dash of salt and pepper. Continue to sauté for 5-7 additional minutes.
Combine ALL the ingredients to the pot with the lentils. Cook covered with medium heat for 25 minutes.
Remove from heat, allow to sit covered for 5 minutes.
If needed, salt and pepper to taste while in bowl.
Serve and Enjoy.

DAY 3
Week 1

1st Meal
POWER RA Smoothie
1 Banana
1/2 Avocado
1/4 cup of Oats
1 handful of Almonds
2 cups of Almond Milk or Almond Coconut
1/2 tsp Cinnamon
2 Tbsp Raw Cacao
2 tsp Chocolate powder (optional for chocolate smoothie flavor)
1 Tbsp Maple Syrup (optional)
1 cup of Water
1 cup Ice
Blend.

2nd Meal
Leftover soup and a mason jar salad.

3rd Meal
ASIAN STIR FRY
2 cups Rice
2 Broccoli Crowns (save 1.5 cups of stalk for day 6)
1 large or 2 small Bok Choy
1 lb. Green Beans
1 Medium Carrot (sliced or chopped. We use a potato peeler)
1/2 Sweet Onion
8 chopped Mushrooms
1/4 of a Red Bell Pepper
1/4 of a Yellow Bell Pepper
Some chopped basil
1/4 cup of Teriyaki or Stir Fry a Sauce I prefer Kikkoman
1 tsp Sesame Seeds
A little fresh ginger (We used a cheese grater, but a knife will do).

Instructions:
Preheat the oven to 495 degrees
Cook 2 cups of rice with 4 cups of water and a few dashes of salt on medium heat.
Chop broccoli, bok choy, carrots, mushrooms, basil, onions, and peppers.
Coat a large baking dish (I prefer a casserole dish) with Olive Oil.
Layer all veggies in the dish with green beans on the bottom.
Season with sea salt and pepper.
Cover and Roast for twenty minutes.
Combine rice, veggies, stir fry sauce, sesame seeds and ginger in a large bowl.
Serve and Enjoy.
*Save some for lunch tomorrow!

Meal prep: *Prepare your granola tonight.*

GRANOLA
Preheat over to 395 degrees
2 cup Oats (I prefer to mix old fashion and Steel cut)
1/4 cup Olive Oil
1/3 cup Maple Syrup
1/2 tsp Cinnamon
1 tsp Vanilla

Instructions:
Mix all ingredients and bake for 15 minutes. Allow to cool and store in airtight container, like a mason jar! (Optional may add nuts or dry fruit to jar)

DAY 4
Week 1

1st Meal
Layer any fruit of choice (we prefer apples, bananas, mango and berries) in a mason jar with granola and coconut yogurt. Enjoy!

A BOLD PERSPECTIVE

2nd Meal
Left Overs Asian Stir Fry

3 Meal
ASPARAGUS & MASH
8 Asparagus per person
5 medium Red Potatoes
6 Mushrooms
1 Veggie Bouillon cube
2 Tbsp Flour
2 Tbsp plus 2 tsp Olive Oil
2 Celery Stalk
1/4 cup of a chopped Sweet Onions
1/4 cup of a Red Peppers
1 tbsp fresh Parsley
A few sprigs of fresh Thyme
1 Rosemary stem (keep whole, use to simmer in the sauce for herb flavor)
1 1/2 cups Water
1/3 cup Almond Milk
Pepper to taste. NO SALT NEEDED.
Plus a Side Salad: Lettuce, Cucumber, Tomatoes

Instructions:
Boil 1.5 cups of water with a dash of salt.
Wash potatoes. Peel the potatoes leaving some of the skin then chop into 6 pieces.
Boil the potatoes until tender (about 20 minutes).
Chop mushrooms, peppers, onions, and celery.
Combine in a saucepan over medium low heat 2 tbsp of olive oil (add the oil first) and 2 tbsp flour stir until smooth. Add 1/2 cups water, stir until smooth and hot. Add another 1/2 cup of water, stir in until smooth and hot. Then add the final 1/2 cup of water, stir until smooth and hot. Next, add the bouillon cube (smash the cube with a fork to mix into sauce). Then add chopped veggies and herbs. Allow the MUSHROOM SAUCE to simmer for 15 minutes.
Mash (with a potato masher or a fork) the potatoes after they are tender

enough to stick a folk through them. Stir in almond milk and 1tsp olive oil. Allow to cook for 5 additional minutes.

Cook asparagus in a pan with 1 tsp olive oil and a dash of salt and pepper cover on medium for 5 minutes.
Serve potatoes topped with the mushroom sauce, asparagus and salad.
(* Tip for neat presentation I used an ice cream scooper for my potatoes!)
Serve and Enjoy.

2 Meal preps: *1st Meal Prep: Overnight (soak) your steel cut oats. How? In a Mason jar or bowl with a lid. Add 2 cups of steel cut oats and 3 cups of water, and a dash of salt, 1/2tsp cinnamon, and 1 tsp vanilla. WHY? It saves us working folk's time in the morning.*
2nd Meal Prep: overnight (soak) 1.5 cups of chickpeas in 3 cups of water.

DAY 5
Week 1

1st Meal
STEEL CUT
Almond Milk
Maple Syrup
Cinnamon
Vanilla Extract
Fruit
Instructions:
Pour the oats and 1tsp of vanilla extract into a pot or a pan on medium. Add 1/4 cup of water (add more if desired).
Cook oats until they reaches desired texture and temperature.
Serve in a Mason jar or bowl.
Add desired amount of almond milk, maple syrup, cinnamon and fruit. (My portions are 1/2 oats with 1 tbsp of maple syrup, 1/8 tsp cinnamon, 1/4 chopped fruit and chopped fruit like bananas, chopped apple, berries and or mangos. Sometimes I add raisins. RA's oats are prepared the same but he add 1/4 cup almonds. Serve and Enjoy.

2nd Meal
Your choice! Be Creative... Maybe fruit, mason jar salad or leftovers.

3rd Meal
FALAFEL TACOS
1.5 cups *"soaked"* Chick Peas aka Garbanzo Beans
1/3 of a medium Zucchini
1 cups Basil
Handful of Parsley
1/4 of a Red Pepper
1/4 of a Sweet Onion
1 Garlic Clove fresh or 1 tsp of powder
2 tsp Fennel
1 tbsp Cumin
2 tsp salt
1/2 tsp Pepper
2 tbsp. Flour
1 Lemon
1/2 Avocado
2 tbsp. Plain Coconut Yogurt
Tortilla shells
Lettuce and or Sunflower Sprouts
1 Roma tomatoes

Instructions:
Preheat oven to 395 degrees. And line oven pan with olive oil.
OR Falafels may be fried with a 1/2 cup of olive oil.
Drain and rinse the chickpeas.
Process chickpeas, zucchini, 1/2c basil, parsley, onion, garlic, fennel, cumin, salt, and pepper.
Once all the ingredients have been processed add ingredients to a bowl.
Stir in flour and allow the mixture to bind for 7-10 minutes.
Instructions: for the avocado spread:
Process avocado, yogurt, remaining basil, red pepper, 1 tsp lemon juice and olive oil.
Use 1/4 measuring cup or 1/4 ice cream scooper to measure. Roll falafels into

ball or patties.
Bake for 30 minutes. After 15 minutes, flip over then or fry for 7-10 on each side.
Layer the tacos with lettuce and/or sprouts, tomatoes, falafels and top with avocado spread.
Serve and Enjoy.

DAY 6
Week 1

1st Meal
GREEN STALK Smoothie
1.5 cups of Broccoli stalk
1/2 cup Parsley
1 cup Pineapple
1/2 cup Cucumber
1/2 of a Mango
1 Orange
1 cup Water
1 cup Ice
Blend.
After pulling into cup, top off with freshly squeezed o.j juice. Squeeze juice from 1/2 orange into each cup.

Meal 2
Mason jar salad or any leftovers.

Meal 3
FRUIT SALAD and Smoothie of your choice.
We are eating light tonight. WHY? To show our digestive system some TLC aka digestive responsibility.
We have had starch-based foods for the past 4 days and tomorrow we will have starch and cheese.

A BOLD PERSPECTIVE

Meal Prep: *Overnight (soak) your* **steel cut oats.** *2 cup of steel cut oats and 3 cups of water, and a dash of salt, 1/2tsp cinnamon, and 1 tsp vanilla.*

DAY 7 "VEGETARIAN"
Week 1

1st Meal
STEEL CUT
Almond Milk
Maple Syrup
Cinnamon
Vanilla Extract
Fruit

Instructions:
Pour the oats and 1tsp of vanilla extract into a pot or a pan on medium. Add 1/4 cup of water (add more if desired).
Cook oats until they reaches desired texture and temperature.
Serve in a Mason jar or bowl.
Add desired amount of almond milk, maple syrup, cinnamon and fruit. (My portions are 1/2 oats with 1 tbsp of maple syrup, 1/8 tsp cinnamon, 1/4 chopped fruit and chopped fruit like bananas, chopped apple, berries and or mangos. Sometimes I add raisins. RA's oats are prepared the same but he adds 1/4 cup almonds.
Serve and Enjoy.

Meal 2
Mason jar salad.

Meal 3
STUFFED ROLLS AND MUSHROOMS
Rolls (2 max... freeze the remaining buns for day 17)
Spinach
1 Onions

2 Tomatoes
Basil
Cheese: slices Mozzarella and White Cheddar.
1 package of Baby Bella Mushrooms
1 cup Seasoned Croutons
1/2 of a Red Pepper
Handful of herbs: Basil, Thyme, Rosemary
1 Garlic Clove
1/4 cups Water

Instructions for Stuffed Mushrooms:
Process croutons, 1/4 red pepper, herbs, 1/3 onion, garlic, and water until dressing/stuffing like texture.
Chop tomato.
Combine is a bowl the bread mixture and tomatoes.
Stuff the caps of 6 mushrooms. Drizzle with olive oil, bake at 425 degrees for 20 minutes.

Instructions for Pizza Rolls:
Cut the top layer of the roll and pull the bread out of the center.
Stuff with desired amount spinach, mushrooms, onions, peppers basil, and tomatoes.
Top with cheese and bake at 425 degrees for 5-7 minutes.
Serve and Enjoy.

WEEK 2
MENU, Grocery List, and Recipes

Dinner for the week
Veggie Soup
Cheesy Potatoes
Zoodles
Roasted Veggies
Fish Tacos
Slaw and Sweet Potatoes
~ Oh YEAH!!!! FRIDAY Game Night/Pizza Party (Team A vs. Team B. We

played Catch Phrase, ate pizza, falafels and salad. We drank red wine and laughed all night.

WEEK 2 GROCERY LIST
Some items on the list we may already have from last week, so check your inventory before shopping.

5 Gallons of Water
Bananas
2 Limes
2 Lemons
3 Orange
1 Pineapple
2 Red Apple (we prefer Honeycrisp, Fiji or Pink Lady)
2 Green Apples
2 Pears
Blueberries (frozen or fresh)
Raspberries or Strawberries
1 Pomegranate (optional and seasonal)
10oz Lettuce Spring or Red Leaf
Celery
1 medium Beet
Carrots
4 Broccoli Crowns
1 Cucumber
Red Cabbage
Green Cabbage
1 Bunch of Kale or Collards
2 Packets of Mushrooms
2 Sweet Onions
1 Red Pepper
1 Yellow Pepper
1 Yellow Squash
2 lb. Green Beans
3 Medium Zucchinis

6 Roma Tomatoes
1 Avocado
Fresh Garlic
Fresh Mint
Fresh Basil
Fresh Cilantro
Fresh Rosemary
Fresh Parsley
Fresh Thyme
6 Red Potatoes
3 medium Sweet Potatoes
Ground Cumin
Salt
Pepper
Almond Milk
1 Plain Coconut Yogurt aka cultured milk
2 Coconut Yogurts any flavor aka cultured milk
Walnuts or Pecans
Granola
8oz of shredded cheese (we prefer cheddar)
Hibiscus Tea (Be sure hibiscus is the first listed ingredient.
Flour
Olive Oil
32oz Veggie Broth
Veggie Bouillon Cubes
Maple Syrup
Slaw dressing (we prefer Marzetti's)
Red Quinoa
Steel Cut Oats
Spaghetti noodles: whole wheat or rice (optional if you choose not to have pasta purchase 1 extra zucchini)
Sun-dried Tomatoes
Raisins
Vanilla Extract
Tortilla Shells (your choice soft or hard. May also substitute for pita bread or no bread)
8oz Fish of choice (Wild caught non-scavenger)

Plant Based Protein Powder (we prefer Orgain. Vanilla is more versatile)

DAY 8
Week 2

1st Meal
GRANNY SMITH Smoothie
2 Kale Leaves (remove stem)
1 Green Apple
1/2 Cucumber
Handful Mint Leaves
Handful Blueberries
1 Banana
Juice from 1/2 lime. (Squeeze 1/4 lime poured into each cup).
1 cup Ice
1 cup Water
Blend.

2nd Meal
Mason jar salad and Protein Shake. (For our protein shake we mix 2 scoops of Orgain chocolate with 1 cup of almond milk and 1 cup of water in a mason jar with a shaker ball per one serving. We have fitness friends while on the go mix their protein powder with just water.)

3rd Meal
VEGGIE SOUP
32oz Veggie Broth
3 Kale or Collard leaves
1 cup Green Cabbage
1/2 pack Mushrooms
1/4 Onions
1/4 Red Pepper
1 Garlic Clove

Handful Parsley
Handful Cilantro
2 Celery Stalks
1 chopped Carrot
1 Broccoli Crown
1 tsp Olive Oil
Leaves of 3 Thyme Sprigs
2 tsp Cumin
Salt and Pepper to taste

Instructions:
Bring the broth and 1 bouillon cube to a boil.
Chop all the veggies and herbs.
Combine all ingredients in a pot.
Cook on medium for 25 minutes.
Serve and Enjoy

DAY 9
Week 2

1st Meal
QUINOA PARFAIT
1 cup Red Quinoa
6 oz. flavored Coconut yogurt
1/3 cup Blue Berries
Raspberries or Strawberries
1/2 Banana
2 tbsp Maple Syrup
Granola
1 tbsp. almond milk
Walnuts or Pecans

Instructions:
Rinse quinoa and strain.
Cook 1 cup of quinoa in 1/2 cup of water with medium heat until water

evaporates.
Cook in saucepan blueberries, maple syrup, and 2 tbsp water. Cook on medium-low, until the sauce thickens (about 15 minutes).
Layer quinoa, yogurt, red berries and bananas in a mason jar.
Top with almond milk, blueberry sauce, granola, and nuts.
Serve and Enjoy.

2nd Meal
Protein Shake and Mason jar salad

3rd Meal
CHEESY POTATOES
4 Red Potatoes
2 Broccoli Crowns
1/2 Package of Mushrooms
1/4 of Red Peppers
8oz Cheese
2 tbsp flour
2 tbsp olive oil
1/4 cup almond milk
1 cup water
1/4 Onions
Handful Parsley
2 tbsp. Plain Yogurt
1/4 cup chopped Basil
Salt and Pepper

Instructions:
Preheat oven to 425
Slice potatoes in thin like scallop potatoes.
Boil for 15 minutes, then drain.
Chop veggies and herbs.
Cheese sauce Instruction:
Stir in a sauce pan on medium heat flour and oil. Add 1/4 tsp of salt to the saucepan. Add 1/2 cups water, stir until smooth. Add another 1/4 cup of

water, stir until hot and smooth. Add 4 Oz of cheese, milk, plain yogurt, basil, and parsley. Stir, then remove from heat.
Place potatoes in a casserole dish. Top with chopped veggies and herbs. Pour cheese sauce over potatoes (don't stir) then sprinkle remaining cheese.
Bake uncovered for 20-25 minutes.
Serve and Enjoy.

**Overnight your tea. 2 tea bags steeped in 3 cups of spring water and 1 rosemary stem. Store in frig.

DAY 10
Week 2

1st Meal
HIBISCUS SMOOTHIE
3 cups of Hibiscus Tea
1 Red Apple (I prefer Honey Crisp, Pink Lady or Fiji)
A handful Mint leaves
8-10 Raspberries
Handful of blueberries
Juice from 1/2 pomegranate (optional)
1 Rosemary Stem (Do Not blend into the smoothie)
Juice from 1/2 lemon
1 cup Ice
Remove the tea bags then pour tea in the blender with all ingredients. Blend and enjoy!

2nd Meal
Soup leftovers and protein shake

3rd Meal
ZOODLES
4oz Whole Wheat Spaghetti or brown rice noodles (optional)
2 medium Zucchinis (or 3 zucchini if you choose to have no pasta)
4 Roma Tomatoes

A BOLD PERSPECTIVE

1/4 cup Sun-dried Tomatoes
6 Mushrooms
3 tbsp. Olive Oil
1/2 Avocado
1/2 Sweet Onion
2 cups of Basil
2 Garlic cloves
1/4 of a red pepper
Salt 1/2 tsp
Pepper to taste

Instructions:
Cook noodles according to instructions on the box, but add a dash of sea salt 1tsp olive oil.
Drain and add 1 tsp of olive oil plus a dash of salt and pepper .
Zoodle your zucchini. How to zoodle? With a julienne, cheese grater, potato peeler, or a spiral slicer. We prefer our Spirooli. After zoodles are cut, lightly season zucchini with salt and pepper.
Chop onions, mushrooms and 1 garlic clove.
Sauté onions, mushrooms, and garlic with 1/2tsp salt and 1 tbsp of olive oil for 7-10 minutes.
Chop tomatoes and a few basil leaves, then add to sauté' to create a tomato sauce. Add 1 tbsp of olive oil.
Cook sauce for 20 minutes on medium-low.
Process the avocado, remaining basil, sun-dried tomatoes, red pepper, 1 garlic clove, and 1 tbsp olive oil.
Combine in a bowl RAW zucchini, pasta and pesto sauce. Completely blend the pesto sauce into the noodles and zoodles.
Add noodles to a bowl. Top with tomato sauce.
Serve and Enjoy.

Meal Prep: overnight your oats...

DAY 11
Week 2

1st Meal
STEEL CUT OATS with FRUIT (recipe listed on day 7)

2nd Meal
Leftovers (slightly warm and Enjoy).

3rd Meal
ROASTED VEGGIES
4 cups of Green Beans
1 medium Zucchini
1 Yellow Squash
8 Mushrooms
2 medium Carrots
2 medium red Potatoes
1/2 Red Pepper
1/2 Yellow Pepper
2 Rosemary stems
Leaves from a few thyme leaves
1 small Onion

Instructions:
Preheat oven to 495 degrees.
Chop potatoes and boil for 10 minutes, then drain.
Chop remaining veggies (save 4 mushrooms and 1/4 cup onion for the sauce).
Coat a large baking dish (I prefer a casserole dish) with Olive Oil.
Layer all veggies in the dish with potatoes and green beans on the bottom, onions, peppers and herbs on the top.
Cover.
Roast for 25 minutes.
Add to bowl, then top with mushroom sauce.

Instructions for mushroom sauce
Chop 4 mushrooms and onions
Stir in a saucepan over medium-low heat, add 2 tbsp of olive oil and 2 tbsp

flour and stir until smooth. Add 1/2 cups water, stir until smooth. Add another 1/2 cup of water, stir in until smooth. Then add the final 1/2 cup of water, stir until hot and smooth. Next, add the bouillon cube. Smash cube with a fork. Next add chopped veggies and herbs. Allow the MUSHROOM SAUCE to simmer for 15 minutes.
Serve and Enjoy.

DAY 12 "PESCETARIAN"

Week 2
BEET UP Smoothie
1/2 of a Beet
1.5 cups Pineapple
1 Lime (juice of... Squeeze 1/2 into each cup)
1/2 Green Apple
1 cup Parsley
1 cup Water
1 cup Ice
Blend.

2nd Meal
FRUIT Chopped or Whole with a Mason jar salad.

3rd Meal
FISH TACOS
Tortilla Shells hard or soft your choice.
8oz Fish
Lettuce

For tacos make Salsa or Slaw
2 Tomatoes
1/4 cup Onions
a few sprigs Cilantro Leaves
1/4 of fresh squeezed Lime juice
Dash of Salt and Pepper

-or-
Slaw: (we prefer the slaw with our tacos)
1 cup shredded Cabbage
1 medium Carrot
1/8 cup Sweet Onion
1 few Parsley leaves
2 tbsp Slaw Dressing
Desired Pepper

Instructions: Mix either the salsa or the cabbage. Be sure to chopped produce for the salsa or shred produce for the slaw and stir in slaw dressing.
After 11 days of HEALTHY eating prepare your fish any way that you like!
Fill your shells.
Serve and Enjoy.

DAY 13
Week 2

1st Meal
ORANGE ZING Smoothie
Squeeze juice from 1 Oranges
Remaining Plain Yogurt
1 cup Broccoli stalk
1 cup Pineapple
2 cup Spring Mix
1 Banana
1 Carrot
1 cup water
1 cup Ice
Blend.

2nd Meal
SALAD and a protein shake.

3rd Meal

SWEET POTATO & SLAW

2 medium Sweet Potatoes
2 cups Green Cabbage
1.5 cup Red Cabbage
1 Carrot
1/4 cup Raisins
1 Broccoli Crown
1 Green Apple
1/2 cup pineapple
1/4 Onion
Handful Parsley
Handful Pecans or walnuts
1/4 cup slaw dressing (use more if desired)
Juice from 1/4 Orange
Vanilla Extract
Granola
1 tsp Almond Milk (optional)
1 tbsp Maple Syrup

Instructions:
Preheat oven to 395
Cover and Bake potatoes for 1 hour or until tender enough for a fork can pierce the potato.
Shred the cabbage and carrots.
Chop apples, parsley, broccoli, pineapple, and onions.
Combine cabbage, carrots, apples, broccoli, pineapple, onions, parsley, raisins, nuts and slaw dressing.
Instructions for sweet potato:
Cut an opening in the top layer of sweet potato like you would a baked potato. Use a fork and mash the potato.
Fill with maple syrup, almond milk, vanilla extract and a dash of cinnamon, a few raisins, and nuts.
Broil the potato for 5-7 minutes remove from oven.
Top with granola.
Serve and Enjoy.

DAY 14
Week 2

1st Meal
Fresh Fruit of your choice

2nd Meal
Mason jar salad and Protein Shake

GOC PIZZA PARTY. It's time to Celebrate; 2 weeks down with 1 to go!!!!
Our group had veggie pizza, falafels, salad and red wine!
Serve and Enjoy.

THIRD NOT FINAL

-GOC this is our 3rd but NOT our FINAL week.

This is just the jump start to our new beginning!

Over these past two weeks, we have had the opportunity to witness our personal strengths, commitment, and discipline to ourselves, our health and to one another!

Foods that we thought that we could NOT live one day without... we have LIVED many days without! It wasn't easy, but we did it! So that, we celebrate!

One decision at a time, we took control of our lives and proved that we are stronger than our craving!

THIS IS HOW WE HEAL OUR NATION…WE ASSUMED RESPONSIBILITY for ourselves, our health, and one another. YES WE ARE our brothers and our sisters keeper too!!!
What we eat affects our mind, body and spirit too; it is time to heal our lives and to spread the word!

Like every other strive, it's mind over matter and nutritional wellness is no

A BOLD PERSPECTIVE

exception to the rule.

As for me and Rashon, we make nutritional wellness a priority because our health matters.
Our greatest keys to success have been...

1. **KNOWLEDGE** we are constantly reading about foods and how it positively and negatively affects the human body.

2. **DISCIPLINE** no explanation needed...

3. **COMMITMENT** to ourselves, to our lifestyle, and to one another.

4. **ADVANCED PLANNING** this level of planning that we have done over the past 2 weeks is not necessary, but it is how we prepare for the week. It saves us from frequent grocery store runs, daily eating out, and over spending. Which in turn saves us TIME and MONEY! We like to win and saving time and money is winning!

We (Rashon and I) love the way that we feel and we know that it is a result of our lifestyle. We experience high energy, clarity of mind, and healthy doctor reports!

When we fall short, (eating an increased amount of waste and fewer plant based foods) we feel it in our entire being, for us it has a several names: Sluggish, Tired, Irritability, Mucus, Eczema, Cravings, Headaches and at times Stomach-aches.

MOVING FORWARD
As we enter this third week of GOC, we will explore what we call "80/20 lifestyle." Allow me to explain this aspect of our journey!

80/20 is the lifestyle that Rashon and I live by.

80% of our meals are *vegan aka plant based* foods and 20% of our meals are waste.

What's considered waste? Food that can or do cause harm to the body.

Our (The Fuller's) *waste* is...
- Seafood: We eat wild caught, non-scavenger fish.
- Poultry: We only eat turkey and it must be organic or hormone and antibiotic free. *We lost the taste for it, but if you desire it, be sure to have organic or hormone antibiotic free chicken.*
- Cheese: We eat organic or synthetic hormone-free, unless we eat pizza or cheese dish out. Most restaurants only use stand quality cheese.
- Bad Carbs: Bread, Pasta, Chips, Sugar etc...

WHY do we call it waste?
Because we are not hiding from the truth. The truth is… those foods create waste in our bodies which leads to obesity, clogged arteries, tumors, cyst, free radicals (bad cells like cancer), etc... AND to add insult to injury All BLOOD PRODUCTS (any food that comes from any animal) carries bacteria and parasites which becomes one with us when we eat them.
NO, cooking these foods doesn't kill *all* the bacteria or parasites. In addition, blood products creates mucus in our bodies (which results in more waste build up and blockage).

Okay, so now since we know the truth about waste, if we choose to continue to consume it, we must be responsible in aiding our bodies in elimination.

The best way to aid our bodies in elimination is to only have those types of foods one meal a day (or less) and skip a total day (24 hours) in between.

For example: We (Rashon and I) may have turkey bacon, waffles and chopped fruit for breakfast on Sunday. On that same day our next meal(s) will be totally plant based and on the following day Monday we will eat totally vegan. On Tuesday{if we choose to} we can have animal products again. So we may choose to have pan seared salmon, veggies and mashed potatoes for dinner, which means for breakfast and lunch we will have plant based meals.
Got it?
*After eating the animal products, we highly emphasize raw vegetables and fruit. Be sure to consume pineapple, it contains bromelain and/or papaya it contains papain. Both fruits have powerful ezymes that help to breakdown

animal protein. Also be sure to eat lots of green leafy veggies because they are high in fiber and chlorophyll, which aids the body in digestion.

A Few More Things To Know...

* When fruits and veggies are cooked the vitamins and enzymes in the foods are compromised and in many cases destroyed. Which leaves the veggies with low to no levels of nutrients. So, if you must cook your veggies lighting steam or saute' them.

* Starchy foods like potatoes, pasta, rice, flour, beans, etc... creates mucus in the body. So be sure to properly balance them with green leafy vegetable. Hence, why with GOC we eat *lots* of salads.
To the point of it all...FOOD COMPOSITION MATTERS and we must be good stewards of our health.
No more feeding our temples junk every day and expecting for our bodies to properly take care of us. We must become our bodies #1 ally!

Let's not negate sleep! It is one of the greatest gifts that our Creator gave to our digestive systems. Funny! But,... Real Talk! While we are asleep our digestion systems are fired up and working overtime. During that time our system gets a few hours of uninterrupted digestion before we are back up and stuffing our mouths again. Upon awaking a glass of water should be the first thing that we consume. Water should be our thank you to our digestive system and with every meal we should drink water.

Let's also be sure to get proper protein/amino acid intake. According to our research, it is important to have amino acids (protein). In the chapter titled back to the basics we give a full detailed list of all the plant based proteins. Over the past two weeks, we have been modest on our protein intake, the focus was to *reset* our bodies.
Moving forward, lets' be sure that we are getting in the range of DRV (daily recommended value) for our protein intake. (There is a lot of debate surrounding the needed amount of protein. I've seen research from 40-70

grams daily. We (RA and I try to get no less than forty grams daily.)

Okay, Back to the GOC Menu.

This week's menu and shopping list is totally different from the previous two weeks.
It is aimed towards independence! We have only providing the shopping list and recipes for dinner. Your breakfast and lunch will be your responsibility and your choice!

BUT- *fear not*. WE HAVE GIVEN YOU WHAT WE HAVE!!!

Daily build your 1st meal around fruit. There is no better way to start the day than with a glass of water and fresh fruit. (We prefer spring water because it has minerals).
Our breakfast is always fruit cups, smoothies, parfaits or embellished oatmeal. Occasional (like twice a month) we have a S.A.D breakfast (standard American Diet) with pancakes or waffles served with a side of fruit, turkey bacon, and/or breakfast potatoes, etc.... with Maple Syrup.
(No eggs for us; we lost the taste for them along with chicken.)

Sorry, if I made you hungry, but this coming up week these things are allowed!!

While moving forward with our journey you can have animal products, *IF* you chose to. Be sure to go for lean ones like poultry and fish. *Remember every other day...*

STRONG FINISH e a s y PUSH!!!

* *Tips*
Be sure to have raw fruits and veggies daily.
Be sure to have daily protein, the most common plant based sources are nuts, protein shakes, beans, and seeds.

WEEK 3 GROCERY LIST

Some items on the list we may already have from the previous weeks.

3 Lemons
10 oz Spring Mix or red leaf lettuce
2 Bunch of Kale (we prefer dinosaur aka Lacinato Kale)
4 Broccoli Crowns
2 Red Bell Peppers
1 Green Bell Pepper
1 Yellow Bell Pepper
2 Sweet Onion
1 Red Onion
Green Onions
1 Cucumber
1 Zucchini
1 Roma or plum Tomatoes
1 Yellow squash
2 Yellow corn on the cob
2 medium Sweet Potatoes
Green Cabbage
1 lb Green Beans
1 large Portobello Mushrooms
1 pack of regular Portobello Mushrooms
Fresh Ginger
Fresh Thyme
Fresh Parsley
Fresh Basil
Dried Cranberries
Walnuts or Pecans
Pumpkin Seeds
Olive Oil
Maple Syrup
Almond Milk
Mrs. Dash or similar

Mild Curry Powder
Garlic Powder
Cinnamon
Salt
Pepper
Veggie Bouillon Cubes
BBQ Sauce (High Fructose Corn Syrup Free aka HFCS)
Vinegar (we prefer wine or champagne)
Soy Sauce
1 cup Red Quinoa
Sesame Seed (we prefer black)
Brown Rice
Black Beans
All Purpose Flour
4oz- Fish or poultry per person (For sliders we prefer veggie and at times ground turkey)
4oz-6oz Fish or poultry per person (For pan sear, we prefer salmon, halibut or sea bass)
Cheese Slices: Mozzarella and White Cheddar
Rolls (make sure it has no HFCS)

GENESIS OF CHANGE
Week 3
MENU, Grocery List, and Recipes
Dinner for the week
Vegan Plate
Black and Gold
Roasted Sliders
Kale and Sweet Potatoes
Quinoa stir-fry
Pan Sear
Big Ole Salad
~ GOC Rocks! Strong Finish!!!

DAY 15
Week 3

VEGAN PLATE
1-1/2 cup rice
1 Veggie Bouillon Cube
1/4 Red Pepper
1/4 Green Pepper
1/4 Yellow Pepper
A few Mushrooms
1/4 cup Green Cabbage
1/2 of Sweet Onion
1 Roma or Plum Tomato
2 Broccoli Crowns
1 lb Green Beans
A handful Parsley
1/2 tsp Mild Curry powder
1-1/2 tbsp Olive Oil

Preheat oven to 495
Instructions:
for my J.O Rice (my version of my Brother Jeff's rice).
Cook rice with 3 cups of water and 1 bouillon cube. After the water has evaporated, add curry powder.
Dice and chop all the veggies.
Saute' peppers, 1/4 of onions, tomato, cabbage, mushrooms with olive oil for 12-15 minutes. After the veggies are tender combine the rice and saute'.
Instructions for Green Beans:
Dice 1 Garlic clove and 1/4 Onion.
Coat a baking dish (I prefer a casserole dish) with 1/2 tbsp of Olive Oil.
Layer onions and garlic on the bottom with green beans on top. Add a few dashes of salt, and pepper.
Cover and Roast for 15 minutes. After 15 minutes, add the broccoli on top of the green beans, then cover again and roast for 5-7 minutes.
Serve with a salad and Enjoy.

Meal prep: Overnight (soak) 1 cup of black beans in 3 cups of water.

DAY 16
Week 3

BLACK and GOLD
1 cup of Black Beans
2 Yellow Corn on the cobs
1 Yellow Squash
4 Kale Leaves
1 Small Sweet Onion
1/2 of Red Pepper
Handful of Basil
Handful of Parsley
1 sprig of Thyme Leaves
Green Onions (as much as you like)
1/4 cup Almond Milk
1 Vegetable Bouillon Cube
3 tbsp All-Purpose Flour
3 tbsp plus 1 tsp Olive Oil
1 tsp Garlic Powder
Salt and Pepper

Instructions:
Rinse and strain beans.
Cook beans in 5 cups of water with 1 tsp of salt and 1 tsp of garlic powder on medium heat for 60 min. Chop all veggies and herbs.
Cut the corn off the cob.
Sauté the onion, corn, basil and 1/4 of a red pepper on medium low heat with 1tsp of olive oil, a dash of salt and pepper for 7-10 min. Save 1/4 of the red pepper as a fresh topped. After saute' is complete sit to the side.
Pour remaining olive oil into a pan and add the flour. Stir until creamy. Add 1/2 a cup water, stir until smooth and hot. Add 1/2 cups water, stir until smooth and hot. Add another 1/2 cups water and the bouillon cube stir until smooth and hot. Once the sauce comes to a boil, add 1/4 cup of almond milk.

Add all the ingredients minus the beans, save some red pepper, and green onions as a topper.
Cook covered for 15 minutes on medium heat. If too thick slowly add 1/4 cup water.
Strain the beans and add all the ingredients to one pot, allow to cook for 5-7 minutes.
Serve topped with cracked pepper, red peppers, and green onions. Enjoy.

Meal Prep: If you froze the buns from week 1... It's time to pull them out.

Day 17 "80/20 LIFESTYLE"
WEEK 3

ROASTED SLIDERS
Buns
Chicken, Fish or Veggies (we had veggies)
1/4 of Red Pepper
1/4 of Yellow Pepper
1/4 of Zucchini
1/4 of Onion
Desired amount Mushrooms
1 Tomato
BBQ Sauce
Olive Oil
Salt and Pepper
Mrs. Dash or similar

Instructions:
Preheat the oven to broil.
Slice the veggies. Add the veggies to a baking sheet (I prefer a casserole dish.)
Season with salt, pepper, and drizzle with olive oil.
Broil the veggies, minus the zucchini for 7-10 minutes. (Be sure to set the timer to avoid burning the veggies).
Season your poultry of fish using Mrs. Dash or something similar.
Cook by searing in a pan with 2 tsp of olive oil. 5-10 minutes on each side depending on protein type and ounces.

Cut zucchini to the likings of pickle slices, then lightly season them with salt and pepper.
Create you sliders. Top with zucchini, roasted veggies and BBQ sauce. (For the minimum intake of bread we will have a double patty, with one bun.)
Side Item: Salad
Serve and Enjoy.

DAY 18
Week 3

KALE and SWEET POTATOES
2 Sweet Potatoes
1 bunch of Kale chopped (I prefer dinosaur kale)
1/2 Cucumber
1/4 of Red Pepper, chopped
1/4 of Red Onion, chopped
1/4 cup of dried Cranberries
1/4 cup Walnuts or Pecans (I prefer both)
1/4 cup Pumpkin Seeds
1/4 cup Maple Syrup
1/2 tsp Cinnamon
1 tsp Vanilla Extract
Juice from 1/2 lemon

Lemon Vinaigrette Dressing
1/4 cup Champagne or Wine Vinegar
1/4 cup of Olive Oil
Juice from 1/2 a lemon
2 tsp Maple Syrup
1/2 Garlic clove (optional)
1/2 tsp fresh Thyme
1 tsp fresh basil (chopped)
Zest of 1/2 a lemon
Dash of Salt
Fresh pepper (I prefer cracked)

Instructions:
for sweet potatoes
Preheat your oven to 395 degrees
Peel and slice the potatoes to the likings of scalloped potatoes.
Place the in a casserole dish with 1 cup of water.
Cover the potatoes.
Bake for 35 minutes. After the time has expired. Drain half the water from the casserole dish.
Combine the maple syrup, vanilla extract, juice from 1/2 a lemon and cinnamon and drizzle on top of the potatoes. Cover and bake for 20-25 minutes or until potatoes have reached the desired texture.
Instruction:
Chop all the veggies.
Mix ingredients for dressing
Combine veggies, nuts, and dressing.
Mix and allow to sit for 10 minutes.
Serve and Enjoy!

DAY 19
Week 3

QUINOA STIR FRY
1/2 cup Quinoa (I prefer red. Why? Texture and Presentation.)
1/2 of Cabbage
1/2 of Red Pepper
1/2 of Sweet Onion
6 Mushrooms
2 stems of Green Onion
Salt and Pepper

GINGER SAUCE
1 tsp of Vinegar (I used white wine) 1.5 tbsp soy sauce
3 tbsp Spring Water
1.5 tbsp Maple syrup
1/8 tsp fresh grated Ginger
1/2 tsp grated Sweet Onion
1/2 tsp Sesame Seeds

Instructions for stir fry:
Rinse and drain quinoa using a strainer.
Cook 1/2 of cup quinoa with 1/2 cup water.
Chop cabbage finely
Sauté the onions (save some onion for your ginger sauce) and mushrooms on medium for 5-7 minutes with a dash of salt and pepper.
Add cabbage and peppers sauté for 10 minutes. Remove from heat.
Instructions for Ginger Sauce:
Combine vinegar, maple syrup, onions, sesame seeds, ginger, and water.
Pour on top of stir fry. Mix.
Serve and Enjoy.

DAY 20
Week 3

PAN SEAR
4oz-6oz of Protein (We had salmon, but you may choose any other wild caught non-scavenger fish, turkey or chicken)
2 Broccoli Crowns
1/2 cup Rice
BBQ Sauce (High fructose corn syrup free) or not.
1 tbsp Olive Oil
A dash or two Garlic Powder
Salt and Pepper
1/4 of Onion

Instructions:
Preheat oven to broil.
Cook rice in 1 cup of water.
In a sauce pan, add 1 tbsp of olive oil with a few dashes of salt and pepper.
Prep protein with low amount of salt, pepper and Mrs. Dash (waist-in is in two days. Salt causes swelling in the waist.) Add protein to the pan.
Sear on both sides for 5-7 minutes.
Remove from heat. Top with BBQ sauce, pepper, and fresh squeezed lemon juice.
Broil for 5 minutes
Steam broccoli, onion, and a dash of salt with 1/3 cup of water for 5 minutes.
Serve and Enjoy

DAY 21
Week 3

LAST DAY!
Let's eat very light, waist-in is tomorrow!

A BIG ole salad with everything plant based!!! Veggies, fruit, nuts, seeds, and as a side item Power RA smoothie with added protein powder.

CHAPTER 5

MISSION COMPLETE

WE DID IT!!!

In the words of our dear group mate SHERIDA BYRD, *Peace and Love to ALL our fellow GOCer's!!!*

THE OUTCOME OF GOC

All in all, GOC was a great success for the Zero Gravity Group! Feedback ranged from new knowledge, increased energy, decrease of cravings, regular BMs (bowel movements), new excitement for life, clarity of thoughts, to weight and inches loss. Sheliah and Artanza actually restarted the meal plan the following month.

The win belongs to Team B!!!

The money ($320) was split two ways.
1. Boys and Girls Club [Atlanta] $160.
2. The Innocence Project [New York] $160.

Team A

1. Sherida Byrd 3 pt
2. Valerie Lindsey 1.5 pt
3. Atranza McGuire 1.5 pt
4. Clarissa Mitchell 0 pt
5. Marcus Mitchell 0 pt
6. Joy Howard -.5 pt
7. Tina Fuller -1.5 pt
8. Yosh Benjamin missed waist-out.

Total 4 points

Team B
1. Shandra Wilson 2.5 pt
2. Angelle 1.5 pt
3. Amour Carthy 1 pt
4. Sheliah Williams .5 pt
5. Melody Gray .5
6. Duane Carthy 0
7. Rashon Fuller -1.5
8. Stacia Rhodes missed waist-out

Total 4.5 points

The ORIGINAL GOC Group ZERO GRAVITY

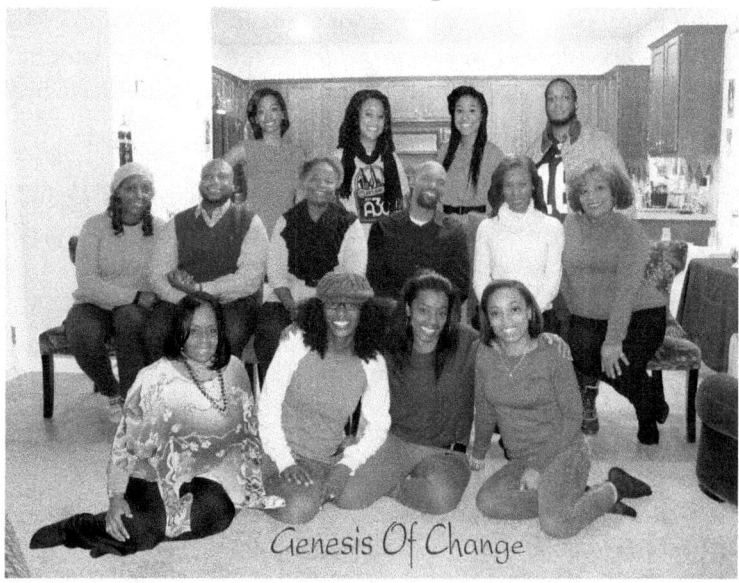

From left to right. 1st row: Mama Val, Melody, Tina, Joy.
2nd row: Clarissa, Marcus, Angelle, Rashon, Stacia, Sherida.
3rd row: Sheliah, Amour, Artanza, Yosh.
Missing from the picture Shandra and Duane.

Feedback from us (Rashon and Tina).

Truth is, we didn't expect to get or learn much from Genesis of Change. WHY? *Because it is our lifestyle, just now on paper.*

Our expectations or lack of were so wrong! Within the first week we felt a new level of amazing energy. Our skin was smooth as silk. Our minds were razor sharp!
Consciousness knows no end...
Rashon and Tina

My big Ah-ha...on the day of waist-out, RA and I both had a waist increase of one and a half inches which was negative 1.5 points a piece. I was as confused as one could be. My mind was full of thoughts...

- How did we flop on a program that we created?
- Our group mates probably think that we didn't followed the program.
- How did we lose weight (*that we had no interest in losing*) yet gain inches?
- I was glad that we were not on the same team... That would have been - 3pts to one team.

First thing the morning after the waist-out, I measured myself again. The day before the challenge my waist was 27-1/2" the day after the challenge 29".

The day after waist-out it returned *back to 27-1/2"*. My Ah-ha moment...Water Weight!
The last night of the challenge we were supposed to have the vegan plate with green beans, rice, broccoli and a salad. Well, I decided to change our veggie. I sauté cabbage and prepared rosemary roasted red potatoes. I only had a few potatoes, my plate was mostly cabbage but both my potatoes and cabbage had salt and it showed during the waist-out.
After that realization I was traumatized! For this book I have moved the menu around. So, now the next time that I or anyone else does this challenge the last meal will be light and easy.

Tina Marie

In the future, when I am 120 years old, still doing crazy calisthenics.
People will ask me, "What are your keys to longevity?"
I will reply, "I eat to live!"
And when they ask me, "when did you make the decision to eat to live?"
I'll reply "My Genesis of Change Occurred in November of 2014."

Rashon Fuller

ACKNOWLEDGEMENTS

Ms. Vera, thank you sharing with me *what God said*. It was the start of a new life for me.

To Ms. Olivette, (*my mentor*) a rear jewel, wrapped in fiery zest, thank you for your life's work and for personally pouring into our lives and so many others.

Rashon Fuller your *LOVE cures my insanities*; thank you for your patience and acceptance. And for partnering with me on this assignment.

Tashon, Jasrah, and Jamal Fuller, thank you for LOVING me and allowing my role as mom #2 to be *embraced*!

LaShaun Lindsey, you came into my world in perfect timing and kept my *heart in this game* called life!

Auset, thank you for *teaching* us how-to write it out and watch it burn.

Melody Frazier and Ebony Mynatt; *Smooches and Love*.

To my Parents Reynold and Valerie Lindsey; my grandmother Mrs. Prince; my siblings Tanya, Karla, Kimberly, Kisha, Shelena and Derval; all my aunties, uncles, cousins, nieces, nephews, extended family and friends both past and present, church members, and colleagues Thank You; for always *LOVING* and *SUPPORTING* me. I have NEVER stood alone, you guys have *ALWAYS* been there!

Bishop J.D Ellis, Pastor Sabrina Ellis, Bishop Eric Clark, Pastor Lynora Clark, Pastors Darrell and Belinda Scott, Pastor Gwen McCurry, Pastor Michelle Moore and to the late Bishop Bill Mikinney, thank you for every word and the all love that was spoken into (our) lives on *that day* and the days there after. Pastor Monique Worship, thank you…

Thank you to my endocrinologist Dr. Desiree McCarthy-Keith, *who has cried in the office with me.*

My *Tiger-Peaches*… I love you guys, Joy Howard, Lakendra Starks and Shelena Omokaro.

My *Beach-Peach*… I love you too Mahogany Rhodes.

A BOLD PERSPECTIVE

My *GA-Peach*... Traci Walker, thank you for encouraging me and showing such excitement towards this project.

Thank you to everyone that had a hand in our **editing**. Your collective BRILLIANCE has given *VOICE to our REASON*: Shandra Wilson, Tamika Jones Longino, Jan Jackson, Mariama White, Sheliah William, and Angelle Jones.

Kervance Ross, [Sharp] thank you for *directing* me in my introduction.

Sherida Byrd, thank you for directing me with a recipe *format*.

C8M, thank you for ALL that was done to make *this book* possible.

Thank you to our team that created a *beautiful* photoshoot: Photographer: Brandon Wigging; Hair: Alkhyseam Watson; Makeup: DeMarlo West; and Wardrobe: Shelena Omokaro.

Ish Holmes, thank you for your assistance with front cover (font) *design*.

Valerie Lindsey, thank you for the inside *pictures:* "Kevin, Grandma, and GOC."

With Much *LOVE* -**Tina Marie**

To my children Tashon, Jasrah, and Jamal Fuller, I am grateful for the opportunity to be your dad; you guys are a true blessing! To my wife Tina, thank you for allowing me to be a part of this life changing project; I believe that it will stand as a beacon of hope for many people!

To my parents Robert Fuller and Sharon Long and to my siblings Lisa Jones, Isaac Collins and Gabriel Fuller, thank you for all your love and support.

To all of my family, thank you for shaping me into the person that I am today.

To my friends; past and present thank you for investing into my life.

- **Rashon**

REFERENCES

Scriptures: The Holy Bible-KJV

Song Reference:

I Surrender All. Judson W. Van DeVenter and Winfield S. Weeden

Pass me not, O Gentle Savior. Francis J. Crosby and William H. Doane

Center for Disease Control and Prevention, www.cdc.gov.com (leading causes of death) 2014

Huffington Post, www.huffpost.com (dirty dozen) 2014

Environmental Working Group, www.ewg.org (clean 15) 2014

Natural Society, www.naturalsociety.com (GMO) 2014

United States Department of Agriculture, www.usda.com (nutrients) 2014

United States Department of Agriculture, www.usda.com (plant based protein) 2014

www.ingramcontent.com/pod-product-compliance
Lightning Source LLC
Chambersburg PA
CBHW062156080426
42734CB00010B/1710